The *Over*protective Brain

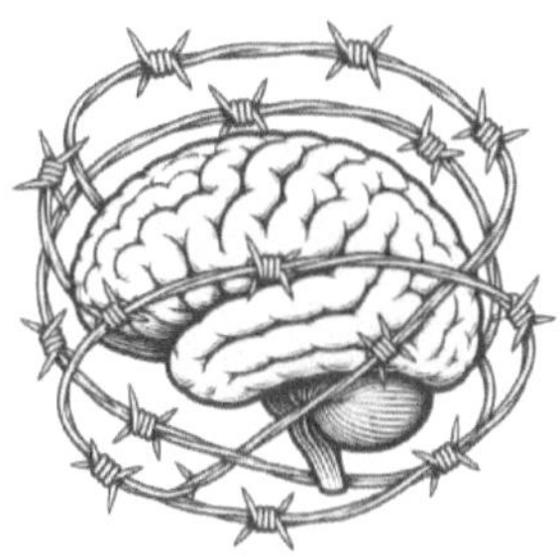

How your brain's attempts
to protect you
are hurting you

Dr. Sam Tyriver, PT, DPT, CWC
Hayley DiMarco

Cover, content, and interior design by Hungry Planet.

For information visit: www.hungryplanet.net

Contents

Preface

I've spent the better part of my career sitting across from people who are suffering.

I don't just mean physically. I am talking about patients who are beaten down to their core just trying to figure out why their body won't stop hurting. They have sought answers and medical help. They have been told "nothing is wrong" or "it's all in their head". Another doctor. Another pointless explanation and more hopelessness.

As the years trickled by, I started seeing patterns. The names, faces and details were all different but on paper, they became the same patient. The more patterns I saw, the more I buried myself in research that was being churned out by brilliant scientists from all over the world. That eventually turned into what we call the Six Keys to Your Inner Pharmacy, a set of practices I started using with my patients, tweaking and refining as I went.

For the longest time, these ideas only lived within the walls of my clinic. They were confined to single patients who could take them home to help heal and regain parts of their lives. One therapist trying to help a few people a week.

It was working ok. People who had hit a wall with traditional physical therapy were suddenly making breakthroughs and finally finding lasting relief.

Eventually, I built the Certified Mindbody Trained Therapist™ (CMBTT) program so I could train physical and occupational therapists all over the country how to do this as well. The Six Keys are real and are helping people, and pretty soon, patients and colleagues started hammering me with the same piece of advice: "Sam, you have to write a book. You need to get this out into the world."

They were right, but I'm a clinician, not an author. A few years ago, I went as far as searching the internet for "how to write a book". I quickly became overwhelmed and discarded the idea because I had no idea how to translate what I did in the clinic onto a printed page, let alone make it palatable by anyone other than a PT or OT.

Then Hayley came along.

She came in as a patient, but she left as the entire reason this book is sitting in your hands right now.

I cannot overstate what Hayley did with these concepts. She didn't just understand them; she lived them, tested them against her own body, and then did something I could never have done on my own: she found the words. She dove into the neuroscience literature with a level of curiosity and rigor that blew me away. I remember reading her first iteration of one of my core concepts. Her words brought tears to my eyes because I had never seen my concepts illustrated so clearly and beautifully. Not only did she understand this material, but she can translate it and deliver it in a way that make sense for everyone and in a way I could never do.

She came up with the concept of Overprotective Pain to describe what so many of my patients feel every day: that your body has essentially turned into a prison, trapping you in a cycle of false alarms. Hayley found a way to translate high-level neuroscience into an intuitive, human story; taking what could have been complex medical text and turning it into something you can actually hold onto, digest and use.

I am a clinician. I observe. I treat. I learn and refine that treatment. But when it comes to the book world, I am a nobody. I am not an author. I can write medical literature or research papers. I can craft an email. I can't write a book that any person struggling with the issues we cover in this book can pick up, instantly relate to, read and apply to their lives.

Hayley can and does so with uncanny talent.

I wish I could treat every single person that is struggling with pain, anxiety, depression, trauma or any other issue. Hayley is the arm that can reach into any home and,lend aid. That gift, which she poured into every single page, is what turns plain medical information into true transformation. I can try to help 8-10 people in a day. Through Hayley's gift, we hope to help millions.

I'm painfully aware that I didn't figure any of this out in a vacuum. The colleagues who pushed my thinking, the mentors who gave me frameworks before I had my own, the brilliant researchers whose work I've spent years reading, and the incredibly brave patients I've had the privilege of treating; every single one of them is in these pages. Science isn't a solo act, and healing isn't either. I owe more debts than I could ever list, and I'm grateful for every single one of them.

What you are holding right now is a conversation that started in a treatment room and refused to stop there. It's what happens when years of clinical observation meet a writer with an extraordinary gift for making those observations actually matter to the people who need them most.

Yes, my concepts and stories are in here, I participated in the process, and I am profoundly grateful it exists.

To Hayley: without you, this content helped a handful of people in Milwaukee, Wisconsin. It is limited to a small number of providers willing to look at pain and mental health with a different lens and refine their treatment. It has limitations and walls.

With you, it's something that I believe is going to change lives far beyond the town I practice in. You have magically made this content accessible to anyone and it can live in every home. With you, millions more people can achieve the validation and answers they have not found elsewhere. This book does not exist without you. You have taken this material and immortalized it. People can read this book and take that with them for the rest of their lives and for years to come.

To Michael, Hayley's husband who edited and published this book and has a profound knack for technology producing our *Overprotective Brain* podcast: I don't know how you two found each other, but the world is better because you did. Your ability to edit this book is like taking a diamond sharpener to an already honed blade. You have made Hayley's unimaginably beautiful words, somehow, even better. You have seen things in this process I didn't even know to be looking for and you know how to deliver it to the world.

To Hayley and Michael, "thank you" is an incalculable understatement of the gratitude I feel toward you and how lucky I am to have you in my life. But I will start there:

Hayley and Michael: Thank you.

Dr. Samuel Tyriver

Licensed Physical Therapist, Doctor of Physical Therapy, Certified Wellness Coach

Introduction

In my (Hayley's) old house, we had a smoke detector with a protection problem. It went off at the slightest hint of smoke. Toast a little too dark, a pan a little too hot, and suddenly the whole kitchen erupted in shrill panic. The alarm didn't pause to evaluate the situation. It didn't ask whether the house was actually on fire. It detected smoke and chose the safest possible response: Fire!

And one of our dogs took it very seriously.

The moment the detector screamed, he bolted to his hiding spot, trembling and unable to settle even after the alarm had stopped. He may have looked dramatic, especially to my husband, but it was just him protecting himself from impending doom.

Then, we moved.

The new house has a "healthy" smoke detector, the kind that doesn't react to every hint of smoke. It hasn't gone off once in the year we've been here. But to this day, our dog still hides when he hears me start to cook. A single clatter of a pan or the whomp of the oven door sends him under the desk in the living room because his body remembers the pattern, and his system does the only thing it knows how to do: protect.

Nothing is wrong with him, at least that's what I insist. He's just responding to the experience he's lived through, not to the new paradigm in which he now lives.

Human nervous systems learn the same way. When something hurts us, our brains remember. The next time we encounter something similar, the alarm system becomes quicker to activate.

Like that time you had food at that place across town, and got sick immediately after. Did you ever go back there again? And if you did, did you feel a little sick to your stomach? That's your brain looking out for you.

Most of the time, this learning is incredibly helpful. It's why you look both ways before crossing a street. It's why you instinctively pull your hand away from a hot stove. Behind the scenes, your nervous system is constantly collecting evidence about what keeps you safe and what puts you at risk.

This subconscious surveillance system operates on what neuroscientist Dr. Stephen Porges calls **neuroception**. Unlike perception, which requires your conscious mind to notice a hazard and think about it, neuroception happens entirely below your awareness. It is your body's involuntary, 24/7 security scanner, constantly listening to your internal organs, scanning your environment, and reading the micro-expressions of people around you to determine if you are safe, in danger, or in a life-threatening situation.

When you suffer from chronic pain or illness, your neuroception has essentially become hyper-vigilant, treating ordinary physical strain, structural vulnerabilities, or minor internal changes as code-red emergencies. To understand how to reset this scanner, we first have to look at the structure it's trying so desperately to protect.

Protection is a part of the reason human beings survive at all. The human body was designed to be a fortress: intelligent, adaptive, and constantly working on your behalf. Every alarm, every protective reflex, every surge of caution exists for a reason. The walls were built to keep danger out so life could flourish within.

The trouble starts when the alarm gets a little too eager. Sometimes your brain can become so committed to preventing a repeat experience that it starts widening the circle of what counts as dangerous, and suddenly a single painful experience becomes a category. A bad day turns into a prediction, and the slightest familiar sensation becomes a warning. And little by little, your alarm system starts showing up earlier, louder, and more often than necessary, and what started as protection slowly becomes confinement.

Most of the time, these extra precautions seem reasonable. Sure, you avoid the thing that hurt you. After all, becoming a little more careful makes sense. So, just to be safe, you pay a little more attention. But as the circle of danger expands, so do your needed accommodations. At first, the adjustments are small. Then a few more follow. Soon, without any conscious decision to do so, more and more of your choices become organized around avoiding what might go wrong rather than pursuing what might go right.

It's like obeying that old smoke detector every time it screams. If it screams over burnt toast, you stop making toast. It screams when water boils, and you stop boiling water; eventually, you will stop cooking altogether because it feels safer to never turn on the stove.

From the detector's point of view, it's never been more successful. Every time it screamed, you changed your behavior.

That's the trap of overprotection. The alarm gets louder. Your life gets smaller. And every retreat looks like proof that the alarm was right.

Eventually, you aren't just avoiding the kitchen; you're avoiding your life. Driven by alarms meant to protect you, your world grows smaller until you find yourself a resident in a prison that was supposed to be your fortress.

If this is your reality, you aren't a lost cause. Your body hasn't failed you. You are just dealing with an overprotective brain doing exactly what it was designed to do: keep you alive. The problem is that it has become too committed to the job.

As a clinician specializing in chronic symptoms, I (Sam) see this exact phenomenon every single day. Hayley sees it under her desk; I see it in patients who feel like they're moving deeper and deeper inside prison walls. Some describe it like living under constant vigilance, every breath, heartbeat, muscle twitch, or sensation examined closely for danger.

If your body feels like this, you're not imagining it. And you're not alone.

More than 51 million Americans live with chronic pain. Millions more experience long-term fatigue, panic symptoms, dizziness, muscle tension, digestive disruption, or other medically unexplained physical symptoms. A significant percentage have undergone every test available, bloodwork, imaging, and neurological evaluation, either to be told that everything looks normal, bringing more confusion than peace, or to be handed a structural diagnosis that makes them feel permanently broken.

When you are left with no clear diagnosis, the search intensifies. You try medications, supplements, breathing exercises, chiropractic adjustments, diet changes, an endless parade of possibilities. And even though each new treatment gives you a sense of hope, like maybe this time we've figured it out, most end up with the same outcome: nothing explains the whole picture. Symptoms persist, and your life shrinks.

Slowly, your body becomes something you must constantly monitor, protect, and negotiate with. But here is the cruel trick of a survival system: the more you monitor it, the more your brain gathers evidence of a possible threat. The attention itself tells your system, "This matters, so keep watching." Once that loop starts, the overprotective brain develops a rigid plan to keep you from future danger.

For anyone who has lived through injury, illness, prolonged stress, or exhaustion, this is what an intelligent, adaptive brain does when it overlearns danger.

But a healthy nervous system was designed to be resilient and adaptive, not rigid. Pain and fear exist to serve a purpose, but they are meant to deliver their message and then stop, not become your constant companions.

When the brain begins interpreting ordinary discomfort as danger, those natural cycles can go into permanent lockdown.

But, unlike my little dog, you don't have to be stuck under the desk. Your brain learned this pattern through experience, which means it can learn a new one.

You can teach your alarm system to feel safe again.

Your Body Is A Fortress

Before anything else, we want to offer you one grounding truth: Your body was not designed to be a prison. It was built to be a fortress, steady, protective, and on your side. When it stops feeling like a sanctuary, the problem isn't a flaw in your character or a failure of your will. It's an automated survival system that has gotten stuck in the on position

Your body became a prison out of protection, not punishment. And because your brain built it, it can also unbuild it.

The goal of this book is to help you see the architecture of your nervous system clearly enough to reclaim agency inside of it. In the chapters ahead, we'll explore a map grounded in neuroscience and decades of pain science to show you how the brain can be retrained toward safety.

You don't need a new body. You just need a different relationship with your nervous system.

If your body has felt like a prison, please know that it is not a life sentence. Although the stance your system has taken is fiercely overprotective, its core architecture remains entirely sound. With a little patience, we can gently calm the panic. Slowly, the alarms will quiet. The guard at the gate can finally step back. Ultimately, the very brain that has been protecting you too fiercely can learn to protect you wisely.

And that is where our work begins.

Part I

The Fortress

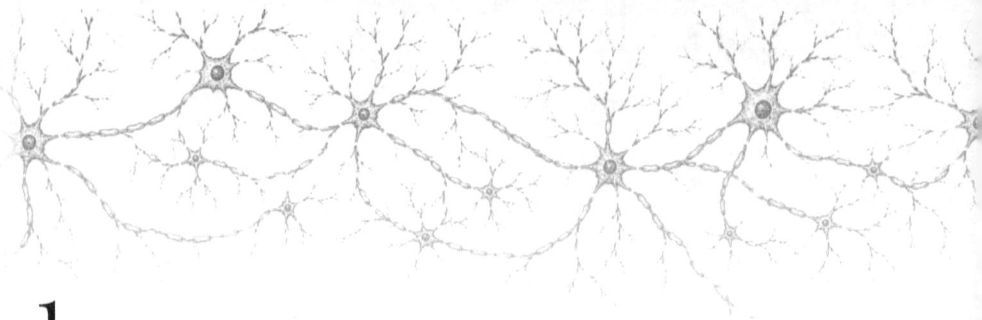

1

The Alert System

How the Brain Detects Threat Before You Know It

"The soul has a thicket of its own because it is a fortress."

—Victor Hugo

Imagine your body not as a collection of failing parts or a machine prone to breaking, but as a masterpiece of ancient architecture. This is your Fortress, a structure designed with a single, obsessive priority: your survival.

Before we can understand why the system meant to protect you has instead begun to pull its perimeters inward, we must first admire the brilliance of its original design. As Victor Hugo suggested, we are surrounded by a living web of nerves that branch into every square inch of our being—an intricate landscape guarded by specialized Sentinels tuned to detect the slightest shift in temperature, pressure, or chemistry.

These Sentinels don't just guard physical territory; they report to a system that continuously constructs the Walls—the moving boundaries of what your brain considers safe. In a healthy system, this dynamic perimeter flexes with your environment, expanding when you are secure and contracting only when real danger appears.

But when the Sentinels become oversensitized, the brain redraws its boundaries too tight. The very perimeter meant to offer freedom starts closing in on you. The fortress, once your greatest ally, becomes a place of confinement. Before we can learn how to push those boundaries back out, we have to walk the perimeter. We need to see how the Sentinels keep watch over the territory, how the Tunnels carry their reports inward, and how the brain decides where to draw the Walls. Only then can we see how a loyal blueprint can, under enough pressure, accidentally build a prison cell.

A fortress is meant to be a safe place. Inside its walls, life can unfold without tension or urgency. Children run around completely carefree. Meals are shared without interruption. Stories drift through open windows. The sun warms the stone courtyard. The air is fresh and safe, because the boundary holds. Safety isn't something you fight for inside a fortress; it's something you inhabit.

A fortress works because it protects what is inside without demanding constant vigilance from those who live inside it. The people within its walls don't think about the walls every few minutes. They aren't controlled by the watchmen. They don't worry about how many arrows are in the armory. The structure does what it was built to do: protect whoever is inside. Protection is embedded into its design.

The Sentinel at the Wall

Every fortress has to know when to activate protection. That's the job of the alert system. At the heart of that system stands a Sentinel, watching, listening, and scanning for anything unusual. He isn't operating alone. Spread across the landscape are sensors and signals. When something unfamiliar is detected, a sound in the woods, a shadow on the hill, a healthy Sentinel doesn't panic or overreact; he pulls the alarm. And if the brain sounds the alarm, the fortress responds just as it should: with proportionate, coordinated action. Watchmen check the gates. Doors are secured. Scouts are sent to observe. And once the anomaly is assessed and resolved, the system resets and peace resumes.

Steady and alert, the Sentinel makes carefree life possible. His role is not to create fear but to preserve peace, keeping out danger while letting everything else pass by undisturbed.

The human body follows this same division of labor. It maintains an internal environment where daily life can proceed with minimal effort or scrutiny by the one living it. When the fortress is functioning as designed, you are its resident, not its captive. Your breath works without you managing it, your blood circulates without a thought, and you can move around the world through a coordinated network that continually balances efficiency and safety. Most of this regulation happens behind the scenes. You don't monitor every sensation or decision because the system has already built-in mechanisms for managing them. It interprets changes, determines relevance, and responds in ways that maintain internal order.

And pain is a part of this protective architecture. It is one of the body's warning systems, an internal signal designed to alert you when something needs attention. Not all sensations carry the same meaning, however, and the nervous system's task is to differentiate them. Some signals indicate ordinary strain or exertion; others potential threat. And it's your brain's *interpretation* that determines whether an alarm will be raised.

Ideally, when this system functions as intended, pain is both timely and informative. By helping you adjust your behavior, it effortlessly protects an area that is healing and prevents further injury. Ultimately, this discomfort is one of several brilliant tools the nervous system uses, a protective mechanism which keeps the body safe while allowing normal activity to continue.

This is crucial for understanding how you experience pain, and before we go any further, a quick note: we will use the word pain as a shorthand for a wider set of protective symptoms the brain can generate. Like dizziness, fatigue, weakness, nausea, anxiety, tremors, temporary loss of strength, and other sensations that serve the same purpose.

Your body is not passive in receiving pain or other protective symptoms; it is actively evaluating the significance of every signal it gets. And that evaluation explains why two situations that appear similar on the surface can produce very different pain responses in different people. Context and experience matter. The brain weighs what is happening now against what it has learned before, and that judgment drives whether your body shifts into vigilance or remains at ease.

Pain Is How the System Signals Threat

Pain's role in the body's protective system is often misunderstood. **Pain is not a gauge for damage; it is an alarm for protection.** And like any alarm, it can be influenced by the conditions around it. A body that is moving steadily and breathing rhythmically sends a different set of inputs than one locked in sympathetic dominance and constant physical guarding.

Your brain doesn't evaluate signals in isolation; it evaluates them in the context of your body's current state. That's what pain is. Not a single signal from a single pain center, but the result of coordinated brain networks evaluating threat in real time. Consequently, biological feedback, like whether you are breathing smoothly or running on the fumes of exhaustion, is woven directly into that split-second decision. Your nervous system gathers that information, compares it to past experience, and determines the response most likely to maintain safety. When action is required, pain is one of the tools it uses to prompt change, slowing down, shifting position, reducing load, or resting.

When you strip everything else away, pain has one fundamental job: to keep you alive. That's its purpose. Your brain creates pain for the sake of survival. And because survival depends on foresight, it remembers every close call, every injury, every moment that overwhelmed you. **One eye watches your history; the other scans your present. It's always evaluating threat, ready to trigger protection, whether it encounters an actual structural limitation or just a shadow of risk.**

And this evaluation happens automatically, without your awareness or control, in the same way breathing is automatic. Like taking a breath, your nervous system continually evaluates the significance of incoming signals, sorting routine sensations from those that require attention.

This isn't a uniquely neurological phenomenon. Across disciplines, perception has always been understood as relational. What is experienced is shaped not only by what happens, but by who it happens to. Cybernetics pioneer Heinz von Foerster captured this idea when he wrote, "*The environment contains no information. The observer creates it.*" That is to say that the meaning assigned to each sensation is unique to every person. That's why two people can encounter the same physical event and have very different pain experiences.

Understanding this interpretive process is essential because it explains why pain doesn't always track with injury. The brain can trigger pain in the absence of damage, or completely ignore a real sensation if it decides the signal is irrelevant to your immediate survival. What matters is not only what happens in the body, but how your nervous system interprets the situation.

The Boxer

A moment that captures this better than any clinical explanation happened during a televised exhibition fight between Mike Tyson and Jake Paul. Before the main event, two professional female boxers opened the night with an intense, high-contact match.

When the final bell rang, one of the fighters walked back to her corner with a deep cut across her forehead, wide enough that anyone watching would assume she'd be rushed straight to the ER. But she didn't react. She didn't flinch. She barely seemed aware of it.

If someone without her training took that same punch, they'd feel immediate, overwhelming pain because their brain hasn't rehearsed in that environment. For the boxer, however, the tissue injury might be identical, but her brain completely tunes out the sensation because it thoroughly understands the situation. Punches land every day in her world, so her nervous system interprets the heavy contact as expected background noise rather than a dangerous emergency. No alarm is required.

Now contrast that with a different kind of contact—an accidental thumb to the eye or an illegal rabbit punch to the back of the neck. Because these strikes bypass her training and target highly vulnerable anatomical zones, they trigger an immediate pause even at the highest levels of the sport. Instinctively, the fighter blinks, stumbles, and curls inward to shield the area. Often, while there is absolutely no lasting structural damage, the resulting pain is sharp, sudden, and completely incapacitating. Ultimately, the nervous system treats the unfamiliar impact as an emergency simply because unexpected sensations are always interpreted as more threatening than familiar ones.

The same brain generated two entirely different responses because it assigned a completely different meaning to each strike. While pain can certainly alert us to real physical damage, it is never a passive gauge; it's always filtered through your brain's level of perceived risk.

The Science Behind the Signal

In a study published in the scientific journal *Pain*, researchers Lorimer Moseley and Arnoud Arntz tested whether a person's interpretation of a sensation could change the pain they felt, even when the physical input was exactly the same. To do this, they applied identical heat stimuli to participants' skin while changing only one detail: how dangerous the stimulus appeared.

The setup was simple. Participants saw a visual cue before each heat pulse. Sometimes the cue indicated the upcoming stimulus was normal or safe. Other times, it signaled it would be harmful, even though the temperature never changed. Their nervous systems responded differently depending on what the person believed was about to happen. When participants expected danger, they reported significantly higher pain. When they expected safety, they reported less. The physical stimulus was constant; the brain's interpretation was not.

This study demonstrated in controlled conditions what the boxer's reaction shows in real life: **the nervous system does not measure damage. It evaluates meaning.**

Your Pain Is Real. But It's Not Where You Think

Before we can understand our pain, we need to dismantle one of the most deeply held and misleading assumptions in modern life: that pain begins in the body.

It doesn't.

That does not mean your pain isn't real.

It is. You feel it.

It affects your choices, your sleep, your attention, your very sense of self. But where it takes place is not where most people think it does.

The experience of pain is generated in the threat detection system, even when the signal begins in the tissues.

To be clear, you're not imagining your pain. You feel pain in your body, but where you feel it is not where it started.

Your tissue doesn't contain pain receptors. It contains sensors called nociceptors. Think of them as nerve endings whose only job is to detect potentially harmful change and report it. Pain isn't something those sensors send. It's something your brain chooses to create when it interprets a signal as potentially dangerous.

In the fortress metaphor, these nociceptors are the outer Sentinels. They stand on patrol, scanning for disturbance. They do not interpret meaning. They just report activity.

Nociceptors can detect and relay only three things:

- **The Mechanical Sentinels:** They watch for physical distortion like stretch, pressure, or strain. When you twist an ankle or pull a muscle, they immediately report the sudden tension or friction in the tissue.

- **The Thermal Sentinels:** They monitor extreme shifts in temperature, sending an alert the split-second heat or cold threatens to burn or freeze your cells.

- **The Chemical Sentinels:** They track molecular changes, reporting the presence of inflammation, high acidity, or a lack of oxygen in the area.

These Sentinels do not carry the concept of pain. They carry raw data, like a motion detector tripping without knowing whether it's a cat or a burglar. Only your brain can assign meaning. Only your brain can decide where to draw the Walls and whether to produce pain.

To say it another way, pain is not your body's broadcast. It's your brain's verdict. A protective call made in real time.

The Body Feels. The Brain Decides.

Pain is not a damage report. It is a protection decision.

The math is simple: pain is not proof of damage. It is proof of perceived threat.

Your brain maintains a highly detailed map of your body, called a somatosensory map. When it decides something is dangerous, it places pain onto that map, whether or not there's actual tissue harm. That's why amputees can feel pain in phantom limbs. The limb is gone, but the map remains.

Pain is where your body meets meaning.

The signals your body sends are only raw data within these categories. What becomes pain depends on how your brain interprets, filters, and prioritizes that data, a process we'll explore inside the fortress of your nervous system later.

What you need to know right now is that nociceptors don't create pain. They don't even feel pain. They can't judge or decide if a stimulus is painful. What they do is generate sensory information, signaling that something has changed. Those signals move through the nervous system and eventually reach the brain, where the meaning gets assigned.

Which leads to one of the most important distinctions in modern pain science: **Hurt does not automatically mean harm.** You can actually have a severe injury with little pain. And you can also have intense pain with no injury at all. The difference is how your brain interprets it.

Hurt ≠ Harm

On a crisp winter morning, stepping into a steaming shower feels like pure comfort. The hot water washes over your shoulders, and your mind sinks into the soothing warmth. It is safe, familiar, and deeply relaxing.

But step into that exact same shower with a raw, angry sunburn, and that comforting warmth instantly turns into a sheet of liquid fire.

The water hasn't changed. It isn't boiling, and it isn't melting your skin. But beneath the surface, your inflamed tissues have slammed down the master alarm switch, throwing your entire nervous system into a state of panic. The thermal sensors in your skin are sending the exact same data they did yesterday, but your brain, staring at a defensive wall that is already under siege, screams, "Danger!" The excruciating sting you feel isn't a temperature difference in the water; it is your brain frantically trying to protect a border that has already been compromised.

This is why calming or reassuring words rarely help someone in significant pain: a dismissive, "*Don't worry, it'll be okay,*" does nothing for an alarm convinced it's detecting smoke. And nothing for a brain convinced threat is threatening.

So the goal can't be to just tell your nervous system that it's wrong. The goal has to be to help it *recalibrate* what counts as danger. And the only way to recalibrate what it counts as danger is to show it a new reality through safe, repeated experiences. When your body does something small and nothing bad follows, your system takes note. Not all at once, but the way trust is built: one kept promise at a time. We will go into this more in future chapters.

But meaning doesn't just shape how pain feels; it fundamentally dictates whether the alarm sounds at all. When the system believes and fears you're in danger, it reacts loudly; when it senses safety, it falls silent. Pain is a vigilant alert system that responds to what it has been trained to perceive as risk, rather than the objective reality of the situation. Over time, this defense mechanism can become exceedingly sensitive and overprotective, magnifying even the smallest, harmless signals into enormous threats.

A System Under Strain

A healthy alarm system doesn't flag every small signal as an emergency. The nervous system routinely notes everyday sensations, like minor strain, temperature shifts, or the pull of movement, and processes them in the background without interrupting your life.

But overprotection develops **rather than appearing out of thin air.** Because it rarely arrives like a sudden infection or a clean malfunction, the process accumulates slowly over time. In fact, long before your system ever starts signaling distress, the groundwork for chronic pain has already been laid.

Under strain for a variety of reasons, your nervous system adapts to its environment. The most obvious catalyst is a significant or a slow-healing injury. However, even seemingly benign disruptions—months of broken sleep, **a long stretch of anxiety,** a difficult diagnosis, or the sheer weight of uncertainty—can trigger overprotection. This happens because each of these experiences whispers the exact same message to your neural defense network: "Stay alert. We can't afford to miss anything."

And your body listens. Because **it can't tell the difference between physical pain and emotional stress,** it treats them all the same way, by staying on high alert. Little by little, it lowers the bar for what feels safe. And before long, it starts warning you sooner, redrawing the boundaries of what feels safe, and turning your defenses all the way up.

I (Hayley) know exactly how this tipping point feels because I spent months blindly running toward it.

Years ago, I created and launched a teen book imprint at a major publishing house where I worked. The project was my baby. I loved the challenge, but it was also relentless. At the time, few publishing houses even knew what an internal brand should look like, which meant I spent months building the plane while flying it. Every decision was new to everyone. Every deadline felt more urgent than most. And every day was filled with fires to put out and problems to solve.

In the middle of all that relentless hustle, I woke up one morning and just couldn't stand up straight.

For a full month, I shuffled from meeting to meeting, literally folded at the waist, trying to manage a massive corporate launch while desperately wondering what was structurally wrong with my back.

Looking back, the timing speaks for itself. The physical lockdown arrived during the most demanding season of my professional life, and the symptoms eventually dissolved not long after the launch was over. Knowing what I know now, the math is simple: my body was carrying the exact same heavy load my mind had been carrying and my brain finally decided the weight was simply too much to bear.

Always Ready

Increased readiness **has immediate physical implications.** Mirroring a deer preparing to flee a predator, your body tightens its muscles, shortens its breath, and focuses its attention as your nervous system remembers everything you've been through. It then masterfully turns these physical reactions into a strategy to keep you safe.

What you end up with is **an overburdened body.**

This is the part of overprotective pain that is often misunderstood. People assume the alarm grew louder for no reason, as if pain suddenly announced itself one morning, fully formed and inexplicable. **But overprotection reflects the burden carried by the system, not just your diagnosis.** It's the natural result of a system that has been doing too much for too long and has finally adapted to survive the strain of it all.

Your nervous system is **compensating. It's tired, and tired systems protect** harder. By lowering its threshold for what counts as a threat, your brain turns up the alarm, completely changing how your body moves and feels.

And understanding this completely changes the story. Instead of seeing pain as a sign that your fortress is turning against you, you can finally see it for what it truly is: **a loyal sentinel responding to the accumulated weight of your life.**

Believe it or not, that reality carries good news.

If we can **get those patterns to shift,** even slightly, toward a more restful state, your system begins to learn that constant readiness is no longer the only option.

As author Anne Lamott once wrote, "Almost everything will work again if you unplug it for a few minutes, including you." It's a simple statement, but it captures a deeper truth: recovery starts when you finally give your system space to rest. When the weight is lifted, and your load can be reduced, your system can recover because it's finally been given the chance to stand down.

Why Pain Is So Convincing (Even When It's Wrong)

But standing down is difficult because pain feels incredibly convincing due to the urgent role it was designed to play. Its purpose is not to wait for conscious deliberation, but to compel protection before harm can escalate. In a fraction of a second, your nervous system gathers sensory input, compares it to your past experience, and decides whether you're in danger. By the time pain reaches your awareness, that judgment's already been made. What arrives in your consciousness is not a process, but a final conclusion.

This biological shortcut is what gives pain its **terrifying authority.** It doesn't present itself as a question; **it arrives as a fact,** pulling your attention with a force that easily overshadows reason, logic, imaging results, and medical reassurance. Persuasion, not precision, is built into the signal itself, since survival depends on fast, decisive commands, not necessarily accurate ones.

Inside your fortress, **these alarms are never suggestions**. The moment the Sentinel detects a threat, your body reacts before your conscious mind can even think, instantly spiking your heart rate, shifting your breath, and locking your muscles just to keep you alive.

This physiological cascade is exactly why **pain feels so overwhelming.** It isn't just an isolated sensation in your mind; it is a full-body mobilization. Because your muscles, breath, and heart are actively participating in the panic, the alarm gains an undeniable power.

Fortunately, this connection is also your greatest advantage. Because the loop runs in both directions, changing how your body reacts can alter the alarm itself. **The moment you guide your body to stop acting like it's under threat, the pain signal begins to lose its certainty.**

A system built to protect your life **will always err toward caution.** It will always choose "act now, understand later" over "wait and see." It's the same instinct you see in a mother bear who positions herself between her cubs and whatever rustles in the woods, charging before she knows exactly what is out there. While this raw priority kept humanity alive long before locked doors made daily life safer, our biology hasn't changed. Only our environment has.

Because this survival response is so deeply embodied, **pain feels absolute.** This reality uncovers one of the greatest mysteries for anyone living with chronic pain: 'How can something feel this true and not be a sign of actual harm?' The answer lies in the interpretation. For those living with chronic pain, the brain has stopped weighing its signals. It no longer asks whether something is dangerous. It just defaults to danger. Pain feels truthful because your brain issues it as a verdict, shaped by memory and fear rather than the actual state of your tissues. **But that authority belongs to the interpreter, not the signal.**

Once you understand this, you can start to hold pain differently. Instead of treating it as a final verdict or a measurement of physical damage, you can view it as a reflection of your alarm's current sensitivity.

Shifting your perspective to see pain as your brain's verdict rather than your body's damage report becomes your doorway to change. You don't have to fight the alarm, and you don't have to convince yourself that what you feel is fake. You just have to recognize why it feels so absolute. Inside your fortress, absolute certainty is what an overprotective system defaults to. But the system was built for something better: flexibility. And flexibility, once lost, can be relearned.

Getting Back on the Horse

The secret to this neural reset is hidden in the old adage, "If you fall off a horse, get right back on." It isn't just cowboy bravado; it is a masterclass in neural recalibration.

Imagine you were once thrown from a horse or bitten by a dog. Long after your physical body completely recovers, just standing near a similar animal can trigger a visceral shift. Feeling a sudden rush of adrenaline, your muscles tighten while your breathing drastically constricts. And before your mind can even analyze whether this particular animal is calm, the alarm instantly sounds.

The animal itself isn't the problem; the real culprit is your body's expanded definition of risk. One moment of genuine danger is enough to drastically lower your defense threshold, causing involuntary protection to arrive sooner and louder.

This is why gentle, safe re-engagement matters so much, like getting back on the horse. In a system that has learned to expect catastrophe, waiting around for a baseline feeling of safety will never resolve the alarm. Your nervous system only updates when the expected disaster fails to happen, like when you actively move, and even if you feel a familiar ache, your body doesn't break down or suffer a new injury. You prove to the system that you can handle the movement safely.

Ultimately, your brain isn't measuring effort; it's measuring consequence. A small, safe movement completed without an escalation of pain carries far more neuroplastic weight than a massive effort pushed through with fear. With every successful, non-threatening interaction, your brain subtly redraws the boundaries of what requires an alarm, teaching a hyper-vigilant system that it is finally safe to stand down.

By contrast, avoidance only teaches your system to widen the alarm; a trap we will explore in the chapters ahead.

Pain is not a measure of damage

Your protective system did not begin life overly sensitive. It became sensitive through experience. What people call triggers are just learned associations; patterns your nervous system has learned to associate with danger.

This is the organizing idea of modern pain science: your alarm is real, but it does not reliably measure injury. It measures perceived threat. And when a system has carried too much for too long, it naturally becomes more protective.

Overprotection reflects the burden carried by the system, not just your diagnosis.

That changes everything.

Because if pain were nothing more than a direct measure of tissue damage, your options would be limited. But because your nervous system plays such a large role in the experience of pain, change remains possible.

Your Sentinel is not your enemy.

It is not malfunctioning.

It is not betraying you.

It is doing exactly what it was designed to do: alert you to what it believes might be danger.

The problem is not that your alarm exists. The problem is that it has learned to fear too much.

Our goal is not to silence the Sentinel or tear down the fortress. Our goal is to help the system recognize what no longer requires protection.

Because a fortress is strongest when its alarms are accurate, not overly sensitive.

And the brain that learned to interpret every alarm as a crisis can learn to tell a threat from a shadow.

2

The Protective Response

When Pain Helps and When It Doesn't

"We are more often frightened than hurt; and we suffer more from imagination than from reality."

— Seneca

I (Hayley) entered middle age with the grace of an eighty-five-year-old getting out of a beanbag chair. By the time I showed up in Sam's office, it was my last-ditch attempt at feeling like myself again. I'd cycled through physicians and naturopaths, followed every protocol Dr. Google could offer, and tried enough supplements to stock a small apothecary. But nothing changed. If anything, everything kept tightening: my world, my range of motion, and my confidence in my own body.

I told Sam during our first visit that I felt decades older than I was. Activities that once felt effortless—walking, gardening, even getting in and out of the bathtub—had become negotiations with pain. My knees ached. My hips refused to cooperate. And the migraines were the worst of it: predictable to the minute, lasting forty-eight hours each time, a cycle I could set a clock to.

After the exam, Sam told me something that didn't match anything I had heard before: there was nothing in my body or my movements that could lead to migraines. Nothing was structurally wrong with my spine or joints. I had no neurological deficit. No orthopedic restriction. No imaging red flags. Nothing in my medical history should have turned a simple overhead reach into the beginning of a two-day shutdown. My nervous system was just responding as if that movement meant danger.

He then explained that my body wasn't malfunctioning; it was overprotecting. And that was the beginning of the end for my migraines, thanks to Sam explaining my Overprotective Brain to me.

The Pattern Behind the Story

Hayley's story was nothing I (Sam) hadn't heard a hundred times before. The details differ from patient to patient, but the pattern is identical—whether it shows up as migraines, fibromyalgia, chronic fatigue syndrome, POTS, or a wide range of persistent, "medically unexplained" conditions. The pattern is recognizable:

- The symptoms rarely start with a single injury.
- And they develop gradually, without the patient realizing when anything had started.

This doesn't diminish the legitimacy of the pain; it just means the system is using a different source of information to decide when protection is necessary.

Hayley's case illustrates the central distinction of this book: Pain always involves the brain's assessment of threat, whether the danger is current, remembered, or anticipated. These are not the same mechanism, but they do influence each other. When these mechanisms are confused, patients can spend years chasing purely structural answers for a problem that has become heavily rooted in an overprotective alarm system.

In the medical community, when any type of pain or physical symptom stubbornly sticks around for more than three months, it is given a broad name: chronic, meaning persistent, pain. But as a master label, persistent pain is incredibly deceptive. It acts like a giant blanket thrown over millions of completely different patients, telling us everything about how long a symptom **has been on the clock,** but absolutely nothing about why it is staying.

To understand why your pain won't stand down, we have to look past the timeline and look at the purpose. Within the world of persistent pain, there are two fundamentally different forces at play: Helpful Pain (The Guide) and Overprotective Pain (The Trap). While they begin as distinct categories, they are not static; under the right conditions, a faithful guide can easily morph into a suffocating trap.

Helpful Pain

Helpful pain points us toward a physical problem that needs our attention. It helps us find what hurts, protect it, and give it the care it needs.

Break a bone, and pain keeps you from using it normally. Touch a hot stove, and pain makes you pull your hand away. Sprain an ankle, and pain changes the way you walk so you stop loading injured tissue to avoid loading it further.

This is pain doing its job.

Helpful pain tends to follow a logical story. Something happens in the body, the nervous system responds, and the symptoms make sense in light of the problem. A fractured bone hurts where the bone is fractured. An infected tooth draws your attention to the tooth. A sprained ankle becomes painful, swollen, stiff, and difficult to walk on.

There is a problem, and the pain helps point us toward it.

This is the kind of pain modern medicine is especially good at treating. Antibiotics clear an infection. A surgeon repairs a torn muscle. A cast stabilizes a fracture. Rest gives an overworked body time to recover. Treat the underlying problem, and the pain usually begins to change with it.

That relationship matters.

When the tissues improve, the nervous system has less reason to protect them. The swelling goes down. Movement returns. The pain eases. The alarm quiets because the body no longer needs the same level of protection.

Sometimes this whole process takes days. Sometimes weeks or months. And sometimes a physical condition does not fully go away, which means some pain may continue to serve a helpful purpose. A person with arthritis, endometriosis, or a permanent structural change may still have a tissue issue that needs care.

So **helpful pain is not defined by how long it lasts.** It is defined by the help it provides, pointing us toward a physical problem that needs attention and helping us respond to what our body actually needs.

Nearly every part of modern healthcare is built around this kind of pain. Clinicians look for the problem, identify what is happening in the body, and treat it. When the condition improves, the symptoms are expected to improve with it.

And a lot of the time, that framework works beautifully, but what happens when the pain doesn't follow that pattern?

What happens when the injury heals but the pain stays? When the symptoms keep changing? When treatment after treatment targets the tissues but nothing seems to help? When the pain becomes far greater than the physical problem can explain? Or when you are in terrible pain and no one can find a physical problem at all?

This is where the second category takes over.

Overprotective Pain

Sometimes, your nervous system produces pain that has absolutely nothing to do with protecting a physical tissue problem. Your pain is not in your head; the symptoms are real. But instead of acting as a faithful scout alerting the fortress to a breach in the walls, the security system itself has become the threat.

This is overprotective pain.

To understand how this happens, we have to remember the golden rule of biology: **pain is not a measure of damage. Pain is an instrument of protection.** Your brain uses pain to aggressively force a change in your behavior whenever it believes you're in danger. It commands your muscles to tense, your movements to halt, and your world to shrink, all to keep you away from a perceived threat.

When your hand touches a hot stove, or when a bone fractures in your arm, that protection is a mercy. The danger and the alarm belong together.

But your nervous system doesn't have a tiny window into your body. It can't peer directly into your spine, your head, or your gut to verify the architecture. It's trapped in a dark room, forced to guess how much protection you need based on the clues it has. For many people, that guess is accurate enough. But for some, under the right conditions, the system begins to tip. It starts choosing protection over accuracy, and once that pattern takes hold, the dark room gets darker.

This overprotective lockdown typically shows up in one of three ways:

The False Alarm: It produces blinding pain when there is no physical tissue damage to protect at all, like a migraine or fibromyalgia.

The Ghost of the Injury: It locks your body in a habit of defense, leaving you in agony months or years after a genuine physical injury has completely mended.

The Amplified Guide: It takes a real, permanent structural issue, like a stable arthritic joint or a degenerated disc, and surrounds it with far more pain, guarding, and alarm than the hardware actually requires.

This is the moment of transformation. It is how a system transitions from one category to the other: a sensation that began as a necessary, Helpful Guide is slowly hijacked by a hyper-vigilant nervous system until it becomes a permanent Trap.

The real division is not about the timeline; it is about the relationship between the condition of your tissues and the volume of the alarm. Helpful pain guards a vulnerability that needs attention. Overprotective pain is an alarm system operating completely out of proportion to the actual state of the hardware.

Once your system crosses that line, pain completely abdicates its role as a reliable guide to your body. More hurt no longer means more harm. A blinding flare-up does not mean a new disaster, and a painful movement is no longer a dangerous movement.

Your brain has stopped consulting your tissues entirely. Now every alarm arrives pre-labeled: worst case.

The Chaos of Overprotective Pain

Because this false alarm is generated by the brain and not a local tissue emergency, overprotective pain completely abandons the standard medical playbook.

If you put five people with daily migraines or long-term back pain in the same room, no two will share the same story. Their triggers, flare-ups, and symptoms will be wildly different because the tissue story alone cannot explain their experience; their brain's unique history is holding the pen. This total lack of a predictable pattern is exactly what makes an overprotective system so exhausting. Instead of following a logical biological path, it behaves like a chaotic intruder:

- It strikes out of nowhere without a clear physical cause.
- It migrates and bounces unpredictably throughout the body.
- It completely ignores the standard tissue fixes, ice packs, and anti-inflammatories that usually quiet an injury.
- It lingers long after a wound has mended, or expands exponentially around a stable, permanent condition.

Just because the pain is chaotic, however, does not mean it is imaginary. You can have an absolutely flawless MRI and still be trapped in agony because your brain is reacting to learned fears rather than the actual state of your body.

This is where traditional medicine runs out of answers. Its injury-based playbook works beautifully when it can find and treat a physical breakdown. But when pain refuses to follow that pattern, you are left stranded.

It is like living with a smoke alarm that will not stop screaming while every expert who searches the house keeps telling you there is no fire.

Eventually, you start to wonder if the alarm is broken. Or if you are. But the alarm isn't broken. And neither are you. The problem is that everyone has been searching for fire when they should have been asking why the brain keeps reading smoke as an inferno.

Why Treatment Fails When the Alarm Is the Problem

If the problem is the alarm, continuing to search for fire will never solve it.

When a smoke alarm goes off because of a real kitchen fire, you put out the flames and fix the kitchen. That is Helpful Pain doing its job. But if that same alarm has become so hyper-sensitive that it blasts at full volume every time a stray dust mite floats past, spraying the walls with a fire extinguisher won't help. You have to recalibrate the sensor.

Traditional medicine is brilliant at fixing physical fires like broken bones, structural breakdowns, and infections. But overprotective pain is a software issue; a glitch in the sensitivity of the detector itself.

Recognizing this changes the entire goal of treatment. Instead of endlessly chasing a hidden structural defect, or trying to aggressively fix a stable condition that cannot explain your agony, you can stop fighting your body. This isn't about repairing a broken frame; it's about retraining an overactive alarm so you can finally get your life back.

When Protection Continues After Healing

I (Sam) once worked with a young woman who injured her arm at work. The fracture healed as expected, and her imaging eventually looked completely normal. But months later, the pain returned with even more force than before. Her arm stiffened, and simple movements felt threatening all over again. At one point, even turning her head made her symptoms flare up.

But there was no new damage. What she was feeling was her nervous system continuing to guard a body that was already structurally stable. She had protected the arm so consistently during the healing period that her muscles adapted to the pattern, tightening, bracing, and refusing to move into positions that had once caused pain.

It's important to note that nothing about her experience was exaggerated or imagined. The pain and her limitations were real, so naturally her distress made sense. Her nervous system had just held onto a protective strategy long after its usefulness had passed.

Cases like hers reveal an important truth: when protection becomes a habit, pain can persist even when tissues are no longer at risk.

When an Ordinary Sensation Gets Coded as Threat

For a lot of us, overprotective pain starts with an association, when a moment that felt overwhelming, frightening, or destabilizing gets linked to whatever your nervous system happened to be tracking at the time. It could be a movement, a place, a smell, or a physical sensation. Somewhere along the way, the system took copious notes.

Your brain doesn't record events the way you remember them; it also records sensory detail and meaning. It notices what was happening in your body and the environment at the moment your distress peaked, then it links those details to a threat. In other words, your brain learns which safe sensations should trigger protection the next time they show up.

Later, when one of those same cues happens, your nervous system reacts as if the original danger has returned. You might suddenly feel sensitive to activities you once tolerated, like exercise, certain foods, or specific movements. The alarm is real, but what it's alerting you to isn't tissue damage; it's a memory your nervous system learned in a moment of distress.

What Overprotection Does to Your Body

No matter how overprotective pain starts, the body responds in surprisingly similar ways. Once your nervous system shifts into protection mode, your brain doesn't just change how it interprets sensation; it recruits the rest of the body to support that decision. It changes how you move, breathe, tense, react, and even spend your energy. These reactions are what a hardworking system does when it thinks you need guarding.

But over time, as you may well know, these responses redefine your physical health. Your muscles become tight. Your movement shrinks, and your senses sharpen. Tired becomes your normal state. And what started as protection slowly becomes part of the experience of pain itself.

What follows are some of the most common ways an overprotective system leaves its fingerprints on your body. Not everyone will experience all of them, and not all of them will feel dramatic. But each one represents a small part of the same story: a system working harder than it needs to, long after the original moment of concern has passed.

Your Muscles Won't Let Go

The most obvious fingerprint of this lockdown mode is muscle tightness. This chronic tightness is actually a defensive strategy known as muscle guarding. The moment your brain senses a threat, even if it is totally mistaken, it locks down your muscle tone to brace and stabilize the area.

In the short term, this is a brilliant way to shield a fresh injury. But when this overprotective loop gets stuck, your muscles can end up partially clenched for hours, days, or even months at a time, and it's utterly exhausting. The truth is, muscles can't hold tension on their own. They don't have a mind of their own; they're just following direct orders from headquarters.

You Stop Moving

Naturally, when your headquarters orders your muscles to lock down, you respond by moving as little as possible. It feels like the safest thing to do, after all. But this survival strategy backfires completely, because movement is actually your brain's primary way of figuring out whether your world is safe or dangerous.

When you consistently guard your body, reduce your steps, or limit your activities, your brain stops receiving signals that everything is functioning normally. Deprived of that real-time data, your system has to rely on threat-based predictions instead. It essentially begins to guess what is safe, and because it is an overprotective system, it always guesses the worst-case scenarios.

As a result, your internal guard narrows its window for what counts as safe. This is exactly how completely ordinary inputs, like a light touch, physical pressure, temperature shifts, simple daily motions, or the stable, long-term structural issues in your tissues, can end up triggering severe, agonizing pain. When that happens, your world shrinks because your brain's comfort zone has shrunk, your system having simply lost its tolerance for everyday life.

The World Starts Feeling Too Loud

Along with restricting your movement, a hyper-vigilant brain turns its attention outward, making the world around you feel incredibly loud. It deliberately cranks up its internal volume knob.

Have you ever told a doctor that light feels harsher, and they looked at you like you were crazy? Or that for some reason, you hear sounds others don't? Or that you can feel everything that's going on inside your body?

You haven't lost your mind. When these exact patterns happen in children, they are diagnosed as having **Sensory Processing Disorder.** But this same sensory overload can easily appear later in life whenever an adult brain starts interpreting ordinary, everyday data as a threat.

If this has happened to you, the most important thing to understand is that this isn't a problem with your physical sensory organs. It is just the result of a hyper-vigilant brain turning its internal volume control all the way up.

Because this is a software dial rather than hardware damage, our goal isn't to fix your senses, but to teach your brain that it is safe to turn the volume back down.

Your Body Reacts Before You Do

Once your brain turns that internal volume control all the way up, your autonomic system takes the cue and joins the fight. This is the command center responsible for your heart rate, breathing, digestion, and sweat.

Because this system is running in high gear, your overprotective symptoms are never just "in your head." They are terrifyingly physical. Your brain can literally skyrocket your heart rate, trap you in shallow breathing, trigger sudden temperature swings, or cause dizziness, sweating, and severe gastrointestinal distress.

These chaotic symptoms aren't a sign that your organs are failing. They are just your overprotective brain frantically rallying your organs into a state of combat readiness, completely mistaking the stressors of everyday life for a life-or-death emergency. These are real, physiological responses coordinated by a brain that is acting as if you're about to go to war inside your own fortress.

You Spend All Your Energy On Protection

Naturally, fighting a never-ending war inside your own body comes with a massive cost: it drains your battery completely dry. Sustained protection consumes an astronomical amount of energy. When your brain is continually standing guard, tensing your muscles, scanning the horizon, it burns through far more fuel in a day than you can ever reasonably supply.

This profound energy deficit explains the crushing fatigue and heavy brain fog that almost always travel alongside overprotective pain. You aren't lazy, and you aren't imagining it. Your system is just burning its daily resources on defense, leaving nothing left in the tank for the rest of your life.

Protection Creates More Problems Than It Solves

As your energy drops, this relentless biological pace triggers a massive domino effect. Over time, the lockdown creates secondary symptoms that seem totally unrelated to your original issue. Suddenly, a full-blown neurological cascade is underway, and your system gets trapped in a vicious feedback loop, producing the very symptoms it is frantically trying to prevent.

I (Sam) recently treated a client who came to me months after a minor car accident, completely bewildered. Her injuries had healed, but she was still experiencing intense back pain, along with, oddly enough, chronic acid reflux, severe fatigue, and brain fog. Naturally, she asked me, "*How did a car accident turn into stomach issues and exhaustion?*"

The answer is a cascade. Because her nervous system was overprotecting her back, her constant guarding and shallow breathing flipped her entire body into a permanent state of fight-or-flight. When your system overprotects you this intensely, the defense mechanism itself becomes the source of the suffering, trapping you under strict rules that shrink your daily life.

Pain Follows the Brain's Lead

This entire cascade happens because your nervous system doesn't just monitor your body; it interprets it. The physical changes in your gut, your breath, and your muscles are all downstream from a brain that has convinced itself the danger is real.

You can see the power of this interpretive process in a famous study by pain neuroscientist Professor Lorimer Moseley. Researchers asked participants with chronic hand pain to perform small movements while looking through magnifying lenses. When the hand appeared larger, their pain instantly got worse, even though the tissues hadn't changed at all. When the lenses reversed the image to make the hand look smaller, their pain decreased.

The tissues were never at risk. The shifts in pain came entirely from interpretation, from the story the brain was telling itself about the state of the body.

When that story is shaped by past experiences instead of a laboratory lens, it creates what we can call the **Rescue Dog Response.** An adopted dog that was previously abused will routinely flinch and brace if a new owner quickly raises their hand or moves too quickly. The current room could be perfectly safe, but the animal's nervous system isn't reacting to the current environment; it's reacting to its history.

This is exactly how overprotective pain operates. Your pain is real, but it's reacting to a memory your system learned in a moment of distress, not to an active tissue issue. What began as a reasonable act of protection has become an old rule that hasn't yet been updated. And rules can be rewritten.

Three Operating Assumptions

To move from mystery to resolution, we need to agree on a framework for how pain works and how recovery actually happens. So, let's agree on three core assumptions. These assumptions shape what works, what fails, and why so many well-intended treatments fall short:

1. Pain is an interpretation, not a direct signal from tissue. Pain is the verdict your brain reaches based on memory, context, and expectation. It is not generated by the tissue itself. This is why pain can appear without damage, persist after healing, or soften when the story the nervous system is telling itself starts to change.

2. Hurt does not equal harm. In a healthy system, pain is just a reliable signal that tissue has been damaged. But when your brain is overprotective, it widens the net and starts entertaining problems that aren't there. Experiencing physical pain doesn't mean you are actively injuring your body or that something is breaking down; it simply means your brain is overreacting to ordinary, safe bodily sensations.

3. Action must precede feeling. Overprotective pain completely flips the traditional sequence of recovery. In a tissue-based injury, the sequence is intuitive: FEEL → THINK → DO (I feel pain in my foot, so I think I can't run, so I don't go running). But when your alarm is overprotective, waiting for the pain to stop before you move is like waiting for your shadow to move out of the way before you step forward. To break out of this cycle, you have to adopt a total reversal of the old order: DO → THINK → FEEL.

The First Hint Your Fortress is Becoming a Prison

There is a subtle but stubborn power in the things we are taught to expect about our own bodies, a reality captured by Frances Hodgson Burnett in The Secret Garden, when she observes that "nothing in the world is quite as adoring as a belief."

In this classic book, we see the world of Colin Craven, who grows up convinced he is fragile, sickly, and destined only to get worse. The adults around him reinforce this idea by treating him like he can't bear normal life. So, he stays indoors, avoids movement, and labels every sensation as a sign of his worsening illness, an experience that started with expectation: his own and everyone else's.

As the story unfolds, Colin's world contracts to the size of his fear. Ordinary childhood activities are beyond his reach, and because of that, his body grows more convinced of its own fragility, having been taught, day by day, to expect the worst. His nervous system, following the script handed to it, says to him, "This is just who you are. This is what life costs you. You aren't like the rest of the kids."

Colin's story may be fictional, but the pattern is agonizingly familiar to anyone living with chronic symptoms. When fear, medical messaging, or a hyper-vigilant brain keeps telling your body that it is unsafe and incapable, a physical prison is quick to follow.

According to the old rules he was raised on, he needed to feel strong and healthy before he could ever dream of stepping outside. If he had waited for that weakness to vanish, he would have died in that bed. Instead, with the help of Mary, who refused to buy into his fragility, Colin started moving first (DO). That physical action completely shattered his old beliefs (THINK), and only then did his body start to rebuild its muscles and melt away the tension (FEEL).

To break out of your own prison, you have to adopt this exact same reversal: DO → THINK → FEEL.

Your overprotective brain is highly skeptical. It does not care about positive thoughts, and it won't be persuaded by comforting arguments. It only cares about hard, physical evidence—updating your internal threat level when it literally sees you move, breathe, and participate in life without a disaster happening.

These safety signals are rarely dramatic. They come in the form of ordinary, everyday experiences: movement without consequence, breath without urgency, and sensation without escalation. Each safe movement is a new data point that contradicts the old alarm, forcing your system to stand down.

This reversal is incredibly uncomfortable and completely counterintuitive. It asks you to move while your system is still screaming at you to be cautious. But overprotective pain is not a broken tissue problem waiting for a medical procedure. It is a loyal protection system waiting for new information. This action-first sequence is how you give your brain the proof it needs to conclude that protection is no longer required, allowing the air to clear and the fortress to finally feel like home again.

When Protection Outlives the Threat

The neurologist and philosopher William James once observed, "The great thing in all education is to make our nervous system our ally instead of our enemy." Pain science would add a vital nuance: your system is never truly your enemy. It is always your ally, sometimes just an ally that learned the wrong lesson.

Helpful pain is a messenger that arrives, delivers its warning, and leaves. Overprotective pain is what happens when that messenger decides to move in, utterly convinced that the war never ended.

A system built for survival does not pause to ask for proof before it acts; it predicts, prepares, and mobilizes. As we have seen, that is exactly why an overprotective brain can lock down your muscles, distort your senses, bankrupt your energy, and shrink your entire physical world. The fortress remains fully intact. The sentinels simply refuse to clock out.

The tragedy of overprotection is not that your system is broken, but that it is incredibly loyal. It continues to ruthlessly enforce rules that were once life-saving but are no longer accurate. The problem isn't a lack of intelligence; it's a surplus of loyalty. The Guard is faithfully protecting you from a version of the world that no longer exists. And because the brain learns primarily through raw physical experience, intellectual reassurance alone can never persuade it to stand down.

This is where true healing radically diverges from our overprotective intuition. A fresh injury teaches us to wait for relief before returning to our lives, and that instinct is correct in the short term. But overprotective pain runs the same program indefinitely. It keeps us waiting for a relief that never comes, because the very avoidance that feels protective is preventing the nervous system from ever receiving the evidence it needs to stand down. The only way to change that is to move before the alarm clears, proving to the nervous system that the body is far more capable than the alarm is predicting.

Your brain updates its internal maps through evidence, not insight. Thankfully, that evidence doesn't need to be dramatic to count. In fact, the most reliable, lasting changes come from tiny experiences—movements and moments that are small enough to succeed, but heavy enough to carry the exact same message: the conditions have changed.

Pain, then, isn't just a misery to endure or a signal to suppress. It's a brilliant, loyal system waiting to be re-educated. The alarm is not a final verdict; it is simply a hypothesis. And hypotheses can always be revised.

A fortress is at its strongest when its sentinels are discerning. Not when they are relentless.

Part II

Inside the Fortress

3

The Inner Workings of the Fortress

The Neuroanatomy of Protection

"The brain is a world consisting of a number of unexplored continents and great stretches of unknown territory."

— Santiago Ramón y Cajal (The father of modern neuroscience)

For most of medical history, pain was treated as a simple input-output system. Stub your toe, your toe hurts. Break a bone, you know the problem. But even before we had the technology to prove it, the pioneers of the mind suspected something deeper was happening. Santiago Ramón y Cajal, the father of modern neuroscience, was not only a scientist but an artist who drew the first blueprints of neurons. His meticulous sketches revealed that the brain wasn't a tangled mess, but a deliberate architecture of individual cells, much like the stones of a great stronghold.

It followed that in the early 20th century, something strange started to surface in clinical records: **not all pain followed damage. And not all damage resulted in pain.**

One of the first to notice this was Dr. Gordon Holmes, a British neurologist working with World War I soldiers who had sustained brain injuries. He observed that while some men with parietal lobe damage lost their sense of touch and temperature, they still experienced deep, agonizing pain. In even more severe cases, where patients had no remaining sensory cortex at all, many developed what became known as thalamic pain syndrome; a burning, relentless agony that morphine couldn't touch.

Fast-forward to the mid-twentieth century, when neurosurgeons like Wilder Penfield began mapping the brain in patients undergoing surgery. As he electrically stimulated the areas responsible for processing bodily sensation in fully awake patients, they reported tingling, pressure, or movement, but rarely pain. It was as if pain had no precise zip code.

By the 1970s, frustration with this inconsistency led researchers like Ronald Melzack and Patrick Wall to propose the Gate Control Theory of Pain, an idea that turned the entire model upside down. Damage has an address. Pain doesn't. Your nervous system evaluates what is happening at that address and decides how much protection is necessary. This theory fundamentally transformed the field, sparking a whole new way of thinking: pain was no longer seen as a signal from a single alarm bell, but as a complex conversation between systems.

When Science Could Finally See It

But the real breakthrough came decades later, when brain imaging using fMRI machines (functional magnetic resonance imaging) allowed researchers to watch that conversation unfolding in real time. What had once been a theory scribbled in margins and a beautiful blueprint drawn by hand was now lit up in color across the screen

Pain wasn't a lone flare in the dark; it was a city skyline at night, alive with signals. Region after region joined in, each contributing its part to the full sensory and emotional experience. Pain didn't play a solo. It staged a full production.

In our analogy, this means pain isn't a single alarm bell ringing in an isolated room; it's a full mobilization. The brain doesn't just flip a central switch; it activates outposts across the entire stronghold. Sensory regions, emotional centers, and planning chambers all switch on in rapid succession. Each area plays its role, in tight coordination with the others, like a well-defended fortress reacting to an incoming siege.

On an average and uneventful day, these different areas tend to mind their own business. Some areas track sensation from your body. Others help regulate your emotions, while still others coordinate movement. There are parts of your brain designed to manage digestion, internal balance, attention, planning, and background maintenance. And under normal conditions, these regions take turns operating. They trade resources. One system moves to the back of the line while another takes the lead. This is how your body stays efficient.

But pain changes both the efficiency and the arrangement, and brain scans shed light on how. Earlier, we described how pain lights up the brain like a city skyline. Another way to think about it is like an old Lite-Brite toy: dark in some places but glowing where the action is. Each region of the brain is like a little plastic hole waiting for a peg. As a region becomes active, it's as if a peg has been pushed in, and light shines through in living color. The more a part of the brain is engaged, the more bright the light. When brain activity is focused, only a few pegs light up. But when the brain is processing pain, it's not just a few pegs; it's the whole board. Sensory regions, emotional centers, motor systems, and the brain's evaluators and planners all switch on at once, as if every peg has been placed, every bulb behind the board fully lit.

This total mobilization isn't a design flaw; it is a masterpiece of purposeful architecture. Your fortress was built to withstand a siege. If a real stronghold is breached, the cooks drop their spoons for kitchen knives, and the blacksmiths grab their hammers to join the defense. The same order is issued in your body. When a threat is detected, the system activates an immediate emergency protocol, deliberately redirecting energy away from daily maintenance to focus entirely on keeping you alive. Memory, movement, emotion, attention, systems that usually work in balance, get pulled into the protective response. That's why pain feels like more than a simple physical sensation. It hijacks clarity and clouds emotion; slowing down your thoughts and fogging up your mind. It doesn't just hurt your neck or your back: it alters the way your whole brain operates. The spotlight is bright because it steals from every other room in the fortress. Why is this important? Because your brain operates on limited energy and shared bandwidth. And when many regions are recruited into a protective response, those regions are no longer available for their usual work.

It's like a video call freezing because too many devices in the house are streaming at once; there's only so much bandwidth to go around.

The Cost of a Prolonged Siege

When a siege is prolonged, the cost is felt everywhere. Digestion, sleep, mood, and clarity are sent to the back of the line, abandoned while the Sentinel doubles down at the front gate. The system reallocates its energy away from long-term maintenance and toward immediate survival.This explains why pain rarely stays confined to a single sensation. It may begin in one place, but it rarely stays there. When your knee hurts, you avoid movement. When you stop moving, your digestion slows, your sleep fractures, your energy dips, and your heart works harder to carry the load.

Inside, the shift is subtle but sweeping. Your stomach stops doing its job properly, and your appetite changes its tune. Sometimes it goes silent, stepping back like a servant dismissed from the room. Other times, it steps forward, pleading for comfort food. And if you're testy when you're in pain, it's not a flaw in your personality. It's your brain, too distracted to keep the peace.

These aren't mysterious add-ons to the siege. They're the predictable consequences of a system forced into protection mode, where resources are rerouted, movement stalls, and the spiral begins. Pain doesn't just hurt. It disorients, demotivates, and, if left unaddressed, dismantles the systems that keep you well.

In a healthy fortress, however, the siege eventually ends. The enemy retreats, the gates reopen, and the emergency protocol stands down. When that reorganization starts to ease the burden, even slightly, the other systems can come back online. That means your clarity improves. Your energy returns in small increments. These shifts, though subtle at first, reflect the core principle of the stronghold: when protection decreases, capacity increases.

If we want to see how this defensive capacity is maintained, we have to step inside the fortress and inspect what each room contributes. Our order here will reflect the sequence pain typically follows, showing the arc of activation, the way a single sensation moves through the fortress, alerting each room in turn, building momentum, and demanding response.

Your Nervous System Is A Fortress

This entire structure was built for your protection. Its walls mark the boundaries of safety, its scouts gather information, and its corridors carry messages deeper inside. Most of the time, this enormous operation happens without you knowing a thing about it. Information comes in, possible threats are evaluated, responses are organized, and when the danger has passed, the fortress settles down again.

The Walls

Every fortress needs a perimeter. Inside is the territory it has been built to protect; outside is a world that must be continually navigated.

But the walls of your nervous system aren't made of stone, and they don't have a fixed location. They represent the boundaries of what your brain currently considers safe. Those boundaries can move. An experience that barely gets the guards' attention one day may set the whole fortress on edge another day, especially when past experience has taught the brain to be cautious.

Throughout the territory, specialized Sentinels keep watch. Neuroscientists call some of these Sentinels nociceptors. As we saw in chapter 1, they detect potentially threatening changes such as extreme heat, intense pressure, mechanical strain, and chemical changes associated with tissue injury. But the Sentinels don't feel pain, and they don't know whether you are actually in danger. They have no access to the larger story. Their job is simply to notice potentially important changes and report them.

Even the Sentinels can become more watchful. Their sensitivity can change depending on what is happening in and around them. When the system becomes sensitized, less input may be required before warning messages begin traveling toward the central nervous system.

Once a Sentinel sends a message, it enters the fortress pathways and begins its journey inward. What started as a simple report will soon encounter a much larger operation. The brain has memory. It has context. It has expectations shaped by what happened yesterday and predictions about what might happen next. By the time that message reaches the inner rooms, it will become one piece of a much bigger question:

How much protection do we need right now?

The Tunnel System (spinal cord)

Unlike a messenger who approaches a fortress openly through the front gate, these signals enter through a hidden tunnel system buried beneath the fortress walls. In biological terms, these messengers are electrical signals traveling along nerves, racing from the tissues toward the inner keep.

The spinal cord is the fortress's protected corridor; a stone tunnel carved beneath the floor through which every report is swiftly dispatched in an unbroken stream. It exists not to decide what is said, but to ensure that what was said gets where it's going.

From the farthest reaches of the body, raw reports of intense heat, mechanical pressure, or chemical shifts travel inward like sealed scrolls racing toward interpretation. At this stage, these incoming signals carry no inherent meaning; they arrive unprocessed and unjudged. They are not yet pain. Only once they pass through the tunnel and enter the rooms of the fortress can they be translated, understood, and given a voice.

Then the traffic reverses. When the brain issues commands, move your arm, steady your breath, pull away from pain, the spinal cord again becomes the messenger's route, shuttling scrolls hand-to-hand back through the tunnel and into action. The same corridor that receives also delivers, forming a bidirectional lifeline, without which no communication could flow.

Without the spinal cord, the body's warnings would never reach the Council Chamber (the frontal lobe), and the final decisions would never leave the fortress walls. It is the lifeline of the fortress, invisible but indispensable, one of two hidden systems buried below the surface. While the spinal cord handles the flow of information, its counterpart, the Autonomic Nervous System, handles the flow of energy. Together, they ensure the fortress remains both informed and operational. In the early nineteenth century, a Scottish surgeon named Sir Charles Bell began treating soldiers wounded in the Napoleonic wars. Musket balls and shrapnel tore through spines, arms, and nerves, and Bell noticed a pattern that medicine had never clearly articulated before: some injuries erased sensation while leaving movement intact, while others erased movement but spared feeling.

From these observations, Bell proposed that the spinal cord was not a single undifferentiated tunnel, but a system with distinct routes, one carrying messages into the brain, another carrying commands outward.

The Generator Room (brainstem)

Just above the tunnel's end, nestled at the base of the fortress, lies the Generator Room, a place few ever notice, but without which nothing else can run. It doesn't issue commands or draft policies, but it ensures the lights stay on. Without it, nothing else could function.

The Generator Room is the **brain stem**, the life-sustaining core of the nervous system. It powers the body's most essential systems, those you never have to think about but couldn't live without. Breathing. Heartbeat. Blood pressure. Swallowing. Digestion. Balance. Sleep/wake cycles. These aren't conscious tasks; they are automated rhythms that keep the fortress alive while your conscious mind focuses elsewhere.

Its prime directive is simple: keep the fortress stable enough to survive. Like the steady hum of an unseen generator, its presence is most obvious when it fails. Neurology has long shown that while we can lose the rooms of memory, language, or personality to injury, if the Generator Room goes cold, the entire fortress falls in an instant. Without this foundational core to hold the baseline, every other room collapses into ruin. The grandest halls of thought and identity mean nothing if the machinery that keeps the blood moving stops. If this machinery falters, breathing ceases, heart rhythms destabilize, and consciousness dissolves entirely. You may not feel the steady hum of the Generator Room, but it dictates the very boundary between life and death.

The Inner Keep (limbic system)

Sensory information arrives at the brain as a neutral report, but it doesn't stay that way. As the sealed scrolls exit the tunnel, they are rushed into the Inner Keep. Deep within these chambers, the scrolls are intercepted by the sentries of the Keep: a network of interconnected circuits known as the limbic system. This network includes structures like the **amygdala** and the **hippocampus**, which serve as a context filter, determining whether what is being sensed belongs to the present moment or echoes from the past.

Your limbic system helps assign emotional weight and priority in close conversation with other regions of your brain.

In these inner chambers, these sentries estimate whether a signal is safe enough to ignore or important enough to move closer to the center of attention. They answer vital questions that raw data alone cannot explain: *How familiar is this? How risky might it be? How quickly should the rest of the fortress respond?*

When something is judged as potentially dangerous, activity in these circuits shifts the entire network into a more protective mode. This is often when survival is prioritized over accuracy.

The scholar Joseph LeDoux, who spent decades mapping these inner chambers, discovered that these emotional systems operate with terrifying speed; acting completely outside of your conscious awareness. They are engineered to make a swift, protective guess rather than wait for a perfect analysis. This built-in bias explains why the fortress can stay locked down in a state of high alert, treating a shadow like an assassin, long after the actual threat has passed.

Helpful pain always engages this Inner Keep to some degree. A hot stove should feel urgent. If you are injured, your brain should care. That sense of alarm is not excessive. It is doing exactly what it was designed to do. But when these circuits remain in a heightened state for too long, the rest of the system struggles to return to baseline; the sentries start treating every minor rumor like an invading army.

Once the Keep has assigned this frantic priority to the message, the scroll is propelled into the final stage of its journey: the high-level interpretation that happens in the Council Chamber.

The Observation Tower (sensory cortex)

Every fortress has a place set apart for watching. High above the inner rooms, the Observation Tower exists for one purpose: to log the precise details of what is happening to the physical structure. From this vantage point, specialized watchmen don't debate what a threat means or panic over its arrival; they simply map out the hard data. They chart the precise location of a disturbance, the speed of its movement, and the shifting temperature of the wind.

This is the sensory cortex. When the sealed scrolls are finally passed up from the lower rooms, this tower rips them open to map the raw parameters of the body. It translates the code into cold, objective coordinates: Touch. Pressure. Temperature. Movement. Position.

The Observation Tower answers only the most basic questions:

Where is something happening?

How intense is it?

What is its shape, location, or duration?

Though the sensory cortex observes the information, this isn't where pain starts. The sensory cortex is just the lookout who sees smoke on the horizon.

But other parts of the brain are the ones who decide whether it's fog, a campfire, or an incoming missile. The sensory cortex provides data, not conclusions. On its own, it cannot produce pain as an experience. It can only report that something has changed.

In healthy pain, the observation tower sends clear, accurate information to the rest of the fortress and then shuts up. It does not amplify signals or hold onto them. It just reports them.

This is why identical physical inputs can feel very different depending on context. The sensory signal itself might be the same, but what happens next depends on which other rooms light up in response.

The Vision Forge (occipital cortex)

In the twentieth century, a man known as Patient P could see perfectly. His eyes worked, his retina worked, but he could not recognize ordinary objects. He suffered from something called visual agnosia, a disorder of recognition. His visual cortex detected edges, shapes, and movement with precision, but his brain could not match what he saw to stored categories or memories. When handed a glove, he described it as "a continuous surface folded in on itself." He could see what was there, but he couldn't tell you what it was.

Cases like his show us something unsettling: sight is not just received. It's constructed. Somewhere in the brain, raw light must be transformed into recognizable objects, faces, and scenes. This construction zone is the Vision Forge, known biologically as **the occipital cortex.** Epictetus once wrote that we are disturbed not by things themselves, but by the views we take of them. As it turns out, our very vision works the same way; the Forge does not merely catch the light, it shapes how we see it.Vision is not a passive camera; it is an aggressive prediction machine. Tucked in the back of the fortress, this chamber doesn't wait for the world to explain itself. Instead, it instantly indexes your past, comparing incoming light against stored memories, learned categories, and old scars.When you glance at a glowing red burner, you don't just see a color, you see a threat. Long before your skin registers a single degree of heat, the Forge has already deciphered the danger. It recognizes the shape of a flame, cross-references it with every burn you've ever survived, and sounds the alarm. In this chamber, sight and survival are forged into a single weapon.

Pain operates by the same principle. Before tissue damage is ever confirmed, the brain evaluates what a stimulus means. Just as we see what the brain predicts is there, we feel what the brain predicts is dangerous. Perception is forged from expectation, and pain, too, is shaped in a forge of memory, learning, and meaning.

But the Vision Forge does not operate in a vacuum. The images it constructs, whether accurate or wildly distorted by past trauma, are instantly weaponized by the rest of the fortress. A single terrifying image forged by memory can send a tremor through the lower rooms, signaling the sentries to double the guard and lock down the gates.

Once the Forge has stamped its visual verdict onto the message, the data is rushed to the highest elevation of the fortress: the Council Chamber. It is there, in the brain's executive center, that the ultimate meaning of your pain is decided.

The Memory Archives (hippocampus)

Every fortress depends not just on its walls and its sentinels, but on its records. Without a detailed account of what has happened before, who breached the perimeter, which routes they used, and what the aftermath looked like, the fortress cannot learn. It can only react. And a fortress that cannot learn is one that will make the same costly mistakes indefinitely.

This is the domain of the Memory Archives.

Biologically, the Memory Archives are housed in the hippocampus, a small, curved structure buried deep within the limbic system, roughly the size and shape of a sea-horse. Despite its modest dimensions, the hippocampus is one of the most consequential structures in the entire nervous system. It is the brain's master archivist: the structure responsible for encoding new experiences into long term memory, retrieving past records when present circumstances demand them, and providing the contextual framework that allows the rest of the fortress to understand not just what is happening, but what it means.

The hippocampus doesn't just store events. It stores the full context surrounding them: where you were, what you felt, what preceded the threat, and what followed. This is what allows the brain to distinguish between a familiar safe sensation and one that resembles a past danger. Context is everything in threat assessment, and context is the hippocampus's specialty.

Presiding over this vast repository is the Master Librarian.

She is not a sentinel on the walls or a sergeant at the gate. She does not issue alarms or route traffic. Her domain is quieter and deeper than any of those posts. The Master Librarian's entire function is to curate, organize, and retrieve the fortress's accumulated history with precision and purpose. When any part of the fortress encounters a sensation that resembles a past threat, it is the Master Librarian who pulls the relevant records, cross-references the contextual details, and sends the historical intelligence upward so the fortress can respond with informed judgment rather than blind reflex. She is the reason the fortress learns from experience rather than starting from scratch with every new signal.

In a well-regulated system, the Master Librarian is exceptionally disciplined. She does not send everything. She sends what is relevant. A record is retrieved because it genuinely matches the present circumstances, not because it vaguely resembles them. Her curatorial standards are what allow the fortress to issue proportionate responses rather than reflexive ones. Without her input and discernment, every sensation would feel equally weighted with the gravity of the worst thing that ever happened.

But the Archives don't function in isolation. Nearly every chamber in the fortress keeps its own personal vault: copies, impressions, and emotional traces of past events. Memory weaves through the entire structure, silently influencing what we notice and how we feel long before we are consciously aware of it. The Master Librarian oversees the central repository, but the fingerprints of the past are everywhere.

This is also why the Archives are uniquely vulnerable under sustained pressure. Under prolonged stress, the doors begin to jam. New records become harder to write, and old ones harder to retrieve with accuracy. Memory fragments. Context erodes. And when the Master Librarian's carefully maintained records become distorted or inaccessible, the fortress loses its ability to learn. It begins treating every creak of a floorboard like the crack of an intruder, because it can no longer reliably distinguish between what happened then and what is happening now.

We see this vulnerability clearly in how humans process high-stress events. After the September 11 attacks, researchers followed how people remembered that day and found something unsettling. Many reported vivid, high-confidence recollections of where they were and what they saw. But over time, those records shifted. Some people came to believe they had witnessed events firsthand that they had only seen on television. Others unconsciously rewrote their personal narratives, folding repeated media footage and later conversations into what felt like direct experience. Emotion stayed anchored. Detail drifted.

Your Memory Archives don't function like a vault with fixed ledgers. They behave more like a living archive that edits its own records, weaving perception, repetition, and interpretation into a single past. This is not a flaw in the system. It is what allows the Archives to update, adapt, and incorporate new evidence. But it also means that under the right conditions of sustained fear and chronic threat, the records the Master Librarian sends upward can become increasingly unreliable, increasingly colored by old danger rather than present reality.

For now it is enough to understand this: the Master Librarian is one of the fortress's most essential officers. Her discernment is what separates a learning system from a reactive one. And as we will see in the chapters ahead, her relationship with the rest of the fortress determines whether it responds to the present moment or to the ghost of what happened years ago.

The Council Chamber (frontal lobe)

Beyond the alarm systems and emotional corridors of the fortress lies the Council Chamber, **the frontal lobe.** This is not a room of command by decree, but a place of deliberation. Here, competing priorities are weighed, impulses are checked, plans are shaped, and words are formed. No single voice rules this chamber unchecked.

Within the Council, different functions take their seats. Some regions evaluate long-term outcomes. Others scan for social risk and consequence. Some support language and expression, while others integrate emotion with logic when tensions rise. Together, these processes negotiate and decide. This is what the frontal lobe does best: it coordinates rather than commands. When the system is healthy, the Council is the ultimate voice of reason. It intercepts the frantic scrolls screaming from the Gatehouse and the Inner Keep, forces a breath, and demands context. It looks past the blinding glare of the Vision Forge and the distorted logs of the Archives to ask the definitive question: Are we truly in danger right now, or is this just an old ghost story? This is the chamber that calculates the true meaning of your pain, allowing the fortress to deploy a measured response rather than a blind, frantic reaction. While deeper systems ask, *Is this dangerous,* the Council asks a different question: *What is the wisest action now?*

To answer that, it draws on memory, social understanding, and predicted consequences. It can slow a reflex, override a fear response, or choose restraint over immediacy. When the Council is functioning well, action is guided by perspective instead of panic.

When the Council falls into disrepair, however, the entire dynamic shifts.

In patients with physical damage to the frontal lobe, knowledge may remain intact, but authority is lost. In other words, the Council Chamber still knows the rules, but it has lost its gavel.

One neuroscientist described a man who could explain, in detail, why he should not eat an entire cake, while continuing to eat it. He could list the fallout, anticipate regret, even narrate his own lack of restraint.

That's because the frontal lobe is where sensation and emotion are translated into deliberate choice. It's what allows a person to think, "*That smells good... but it's not mine, so I won't grab it and eat it.*" Not because you don't want it, but because the long-term costs matter. The Council keeps the future in view.

In this way, the frontal lobe creates space between your desires and your decisions. That's the space for wisdom, and it allows the fortress to protect not only your survival, but your relationships, sense of timing, and your longterm wellbeing.

The Dispatch Hall (primary motor cortex)

High in the fortress, the Dispatch Hall serves as the launch point for every voluntary action we take, from lifting a hand to writing a sentence. Neurobiologically, this is the **primary motor cortex,** a narrow band of tissue running like a headband across the top of the brain. Though compact in shape, it holds a sweeping map of the body, with each section corresponding to a specific region: fingers, toes, face, limbs. This topographical layout is often called **the motor homunculus**: a distorted body sculpted by control rather than size.

The Dispatch Hall is not just a map, though; it is a chamber of orchestration. This is where intention becomes motion. Signals arrive here already shaped by higher-order processing, by evaluation, context, and internal goals, and are converted into precise motor commands. The role of the Dispatch Hall is not to debate or interpret those signals, but to issue them efficiently.

From this room, instructions are sent outward through established routes, carried rapidly along descending pathways into the spinal cord and on to the muscles. Neurons act like mounted messengers, traveling well-worn roads toward specific destinations. At their arrival, fingers curve into a grip, legs stride forward, and the chest deepens its breath. Action unfolds not as a blind reflex, but as a deliberate choice translated into movement.

This room captures the transition from decision to doing. It's where thought becomes action. If the frontal lobe is the strategy room, the Dispatch Hall is the staging ground; full of motion, urgency, and specificity. Damage here does not impair thought or intent, but can paralyze action. It is a reminder that what we choose is not always what we enact, and that even the best plans need a functional dispatch to be carried out.

Coordination Matters More Than Any Single Room

We have walked the winding corridors of the fortress, from the deep dark of the entry tunnels to the high elevation of the executive chambers. We have seen how each room operates, how the sentries watch the gates, and how the scribes edit the past. But to truly understand pain, we have to stop looking at the individual rooms and look at the fortress as a whole.

Pain is not a single alarm being set off in a lone, isolated tower; it is a full mobilization of the stronghold. The Sentinel doesn't just flip a central switch; he activates every outpost across the structure simultaneously. Pain is born from this frantic interaction—a system-wide negotiation deciding what matters in the face of an incoming siege.

- **The Walls (tissue):** register the initial breach and send the first warning message inward.

- **The Tunnel System (spinal cord):** sends those raw signals up from the outer borders.

- **The Generator Room (brainstem):** fuels the system with arousal, vigilance, and raw power.

- **The Inner Keep (limbic system):** assigns urgency, flooding the corridors with raw emotion.

- **The Observation Tower (sensory cortex):** maps the physical location, measuring exactly where it hurts.

- **The Vision Forge (occipital cortex):** decodes the surroundings and shapes what we expect to see.

- **The Memory Archives (hippocampus):** consults historical logs for past context and meaning.

- **The Council Chamber (frontal lobe):** deliberates, weighs consequences, and organizes the final decision.

- **The Dispatch Hall (primary motor cortex):** converts those decisions into immediate, coordinated action.

When these systems communicate clearly and stand down appropriately, pain fulfills its purpose. It alerts, guides, and resolves.

But the system does not always march in that tidy order.

Sometimes the alarm refuses to wait for deliberation. When a signal is tagged with pure, blinding urgency, it takes an emergency bypass, triggering physical action before you've had time to think. This is why your body can flinch, strike, or flee before your conscious mind even registers the threat. The high peak of the Council Chamber still sits at the top of the fortress, but it is entirely bypassed in the name of raw speed.

And when this internal communication breaks down, when the pathways become permanently biased toward danger, the exact same architecture produces a terrifyingly different experience.

Why This Matters Before We Go Further

Understanding the interior of the fortress sets the stage for everything that follows. Pain is not a structural flaw in one isolated room of the brain; it's the collective result of a system doing exactly what it was designed to do. Every single outpost, whether scanning, sensing, deciding, remembering, or commanding plays a vital role in keeping you alive.

Meaning depends entirely on this internal coordination. A single warning scroll from the borders can feel like a catastrophic crisis if the Council panics, or it can fade into background noise if they cue restraint.

That's why mapping this architecture matters so much. We aren't just dealing with raw, mechanical pain signals; we are navigating a complex network of communication and interpretation. Your brain isn't just a passive witness to pain; it determines how that pain is interpreted and expressed. That is why the exact same physical signal can be treated as completely safe or deeply threatening, depending entirely on how your system reads the room.

None of this is set in stone. The fortress learns, changes, and absorbs the impact of everything you've been through. That means true safety isn't just about who is knocking at the outer gates right now; it's about the ghosts the fortress expects to see. Sometimes, the fortress has a perfectly good reason to lock down. Other times, it is simply haunted by the last siege. In those moments, it becomes suffocatingly overprotective in the name of keeping you from sieges past.

When the stronghold is doing its job well, you won't even notice it working. The sentries spot trouble, handle it quietly at the gates, and never bother the rest of the castle with the details. Pain does exactly what it's supposed to do—it shows up to warn you, finishes its job, and leaves. The Sentinels file their reports, step back from the parapets, and rest.

But when the fortress learns to expect danger at every turn, it starts overreacting to everyday sensations. A normal amount of physical strain gets treated like a violent breach, and a random shadow outside the walls feels like a hostile assassin searching for an unlocked gate. The stronghold stops responding to what is actually happening outside and starts reacting to its own worst-case scenarios. Before we can talk about how to calm everything down, we have to understand exactly what the fortress is trying to protect and how it got so turned around in the first place.

In the chapters ahead, we will walk through this process of perception and protection in close detail. We will explore how information flows through these corridors, how gates slam shut, how messengers get intercepted, and how the system decides what finally reaches your conscious awareness. We'll look at what happens when prediction completely replaces perception, and the brain no longer waits to be alarmed, but assumes it should stay on high alert.

We will also uncover why some Sentinels never stand down, even years after the danger has passed, and how painful memories can physically reshape the blueprint of the entire castle.

But for now, it is enough to understand this: Pain is not one single room. It is the whole fortress responding in sync. And when that response no longer matches reality, the first step toward change is not attempting to remove pain; it is learning how your unique system functions.

4

Tunnel Checkpoints

How Pain Moves through the Brain

"Everything was beautiful, and nothing hurt."

— *Kurt Vonnegut, Slaughterhouse-Five*

A fortress is only as safe as its entryways. We already know that signals from the perimeter have to travel through the Tunnel System (the spinal cord) to reach the brain. But these tunnels aren't wide-open highways; they are heavily regulated. They determine who gets through to the inner keep and who gets turned away.

When heat rises, pressure increases, or your chemistry changes, your nerve endings (the Sentries) register the disturbance and dispatch electrical signals toward the brain. But that change is not yet pain. It is not even necessarily danger. It's just a signal picked up by receptors at the perimeter of your body. Before that scroll can ever reach conscious awareness, it has to pass through a regulatory checkpoint inside the Tunnel System, a mechanical gate that can slide shut at a moment's notice.

The speed of these messages is critical because it determines who arrives at the checkpoint first. Your nervous system has an express lane for certain types of information: the safe sensations of touch, movement, and vibration. These safe messages travel on thick, insulated nerve fibers at lightning speed.

The messages of potential danger, however, are relegated to the slow lane. They travel on thin, uninsulated wires, crawling toward the spine at a fraction of the speed of those safe sensations. Whether they are allowed to pass through the tunnel and reach the brain depends entirely on what happens when they hit that checkpoint.

When Things Heat Up

Imagine you are cooking dinner, distracted by a conversation, and your hand brushes the edge of a hot stove.

In an instant, your entire world narrows to that sensation. You flinch, you yelp, and a searing heat radiates up your arm. It feels like an immediate, full-body sensation. But while it feels instantaneous, your nervous system just performed a high-speed triage.

The heat message was prioritized and allowed to rush straight through the checkpoint. Most everyday messages don't get that kind of clearance. At any given second, your body is sending thousands of routine scrolls up the tunnels: the texture of the kitchen floor under your feet, the rhythm of your breathing, the weight of the apron against your waist. You aren't in agony from your clothes because the tunnel checkpoint is closed to those routine updates. They are permanently filtered out as harmless background noise, ensuring the brain isn't overwhelmed by the mundane reality of just existing.

Pain is not just a signal being sent; it is the result of that signal being granted entry to your conscious mind.

The Tunnel System

This constant, around-the-clock filtering is the secret mechanism inside those individual cells Santiago Ramón y Cajal first sketched. For generations after his blueprints, medicine still clung to that simple input-output model, treating the spinal cord like a passive cable, a direct, unthinking wire.

But in the 1960s, researchers Ronald Melzack and Patrick Wall realized the math still didn't add up. They leaned on glaring contradictions that the old model couldn't explain: soldiers on battlefields with massive wounds who felt entirely fine, or patients with minor scratches experiencing agonizing pain.

Their breakthrough discovery changed everything. They proved that the Tunnel System (the spinal cord) isn't just a passive passageway; it is a sophisticated processing center with its own independent regulatory crew.

They called this Gate Control Theory, revealing that the spinal cord acts as a series of heavy checkpoints built into every single segment of your spine. These checkpoints have the power to completely block a warning scroll or radically amplify it before it ever continues its journey up toward the Gatehouse (the thalamus), the brain's central relay station. Think of the Tunnel System like a high-security transit line.

The Entry Checkpoint: When you stub your toe, that warning scroll enters the Tunnel System at the very lowest level of your spine. It has to clear the checkpoint at that exact basement gate just to begin its long journey up toward the brain.

The Corridor Inspection: As the message travels up the Tunnel, it passes through various checkpoints along the way, and at every single level, the system re-evaluates the situation: *Is this scroll still urgent? Has a more critical message arrived from somewhere else that needs to take priority?*

The Gatehouse Clearance: Only after surviving this gauntlet of inspections does the warning scroll finally emerge from the tunnels and reach the Gatehouse (the thalamus), where it can be prepared for the Council up in the brain.

By transforming the spinal cord from a passive cable into a high-security checkpoint, Melzack and Wall completely rewrote our understanding of how data reaches our conscious awareness.

Noise vs. News

To trace exactly how the system negotiates these boundaries, we have to look at the traffic laws of the spinal cord, which serve as a natural filter dividing ordinary environmental noise from breaking survival news.

In the world of medicine, triage is the high-stakes process of sorting. If you walk into a busy emergency room with a life-threatening wound, the triage nurse moves you straight to the front of the line. If you walk in with a mild cough, you are asked to take a seat in the lobby. Your spinal cord performs this same service for the millions of signals flooding in from your body every second.

Once a message enters the Tunnel System at its local gateway, it doesn't just get a free ride to the top. From that entry point onward, the message must clear another checkpoint at every single segment of the tunnel it passes through on its way up to the brain. This triage is the only thing standing between you and absolute sensory chaos. Your nervous system has a bandwidth problem: your conscious mind can only process a fraction of what your body experiences. If every single sensation, the weight of your watch, the temperature of the air, the texture of your socks, reached your brain at once, you would be paralyzed by the sheer noise of it all. The Triage Corridor is the filter that ensures that background hum stays silent while the breaking news gets an express pass to the top.

Winning the Duel

The reason researchers Melzack and Wall called it a gate is because the system can literally shut the gate on a message before it ever reaches your awareness.

For decades, we believed the body was wired like a lamp; flip the switch at one end, and the light must come on at the other. But Melzack and Wall proved that the spinal cord isn't a wire; it's a gatekeeper. By proving that the sensory signals could physically block the danger signals, they showed that the body has the power to silence a signal before the brain ever hears it.

To understand how this works, we have to look at the two types of lanes involved:

- **The Slow Lane (C-Fibers)**: These carry the deep, aching signals of a bumped elbow or a twisted ankle. They are thin and unshielded, meaning the signal crawls along at less than 2 miles per hour.
- **The Express Lane (A-Beta Fibers)**: These carry sensations of touch, vibration, and pressure. They are thick and heavily insulated, allowing signals to travel at a blistering 250 miles per hour.

When you bump your funny bone, those slow-lane signals start their trek toward the brain. If you do nothing, they reach the gate in the spinal cord, pass through, and you feel the full, throbbing sting. But you instinctively rub your elbow or shake out your wrist. This is a biological jamming. By rubbing or shaking, you flood the nervous system with fast-path signals of vibration and pressure. In neuroscience, this is called inhibition. Because these express-lane signals are thousands of times faster, they occupy the gate's capacity, effectively closing it to the slower pain signals trailing behind.

The Power of Vibration

Researchers have found that high-frequency vibration can reduce clinical pain by up to 40%. This is the signal competition in action. By activating the large-diameter nerve fibers (the high-speed A-Beta fibers), the vibration creates so much sensory input that the nociceptive (danger) signals just can't get through the neurological gate.

This is why doctors now use vibrating tools to numb the skin before giving a needle; they are temporarily crowding the gate with movement. Many dentists use a tool called a DentalVibe to vibrate the gums while they inject the local anesthetic so the patient never feels the pinch.

This concept explains why your percussion massage gun can feel so good. The rapid, rhythmic pulses don't necessarily change the tissue beneath it. What it changes is the sensory landscape. By saturating the nervous system with fast, predictable input, it inhibits the pain response and creates the unmistakable sensation of relief.

The Sergeant of the Gate

Any message that successfully fights its way through the entire length of the Triage Corridor finally emerges at the base of the brain. Here, at the top of the spinal tunnels, sits the Gatehouse (the thalamus).

To truly appreciate this space, it helps to understand the sheer scale of the data being managed. At any given millisecond, your body is a literal library of information, an archive that never stops growing. Every hair follicle that moves in the breeze, every joint that carries your weight, and every internal organ doing its slow, rhythmic work is sending a sensory report forward.

Imagine thousands of sensors, scattered from your scalp to your toenails, each frantically filing updates about the world around them:

- One sensor is documenting the exact milligram of pressure from your watch strap against your wrist.
- Another is logging the one-degree shift in the air temperature near your ankle.
- A hundred more are submitting updates on the precise tension in your calf muscles as you shift your weight.

If all of this reached your conscious mind at once, you wouldn't be able to think, speak, or function. You would be completely paralyzed by a sensory flood; a white noise of the body so loud it would drown out the world outside.This is where the Sergeant of the Gate steps in. Stationed at his post inside the Gatehouse, his job is not to just watch the incoming traffic pass through. He screens it. He treats your body's sensory input like an endless stream of incoming dispatches, but he is far too seasoned to be derailed by routine reports. As the senior officer at your nervous system's filtering post, he holds the repetitive reports from your joints and skin at the gate, keeping the lines clear and the fortress uncluttered. Only when something truly urgent arrives, like a sharp sting or a sudden burn, does he wave it through with full priority clearance and send it straight to your conscious command.

The Three Laws of the Gatehouse

To keep this massive archive under control, the Sergeant of the Gate runs his gatehouse desk like a high-stakes newsroom, relying on three strict biological laws to decide what is dropped on the floor as background noise, and what is broadcast to the high towers of your conscious mind as breaking news.

1. The Law of Novelty (The Search for a Scoop)

Your nervous system is tuned entirely to novelty. It is designed to detect change, not static states. If a message stays the same for a long time, like the pressure of the chair you've been sitting in for the last twenty minutes, that's considered old news, and your nerves stop reporting it so aggressively. This is why you can lose your glasses on top of your own head until someone points them out. Your system has triaged that information as static. The data is still there, but it's no longer important enough to make the front page of your conscious mind.

2. The Law of Contrast (The Bold Headline)

While the Law of Novelty actively buries old stories over time, the Law of Contrast is how a message forces its way past that time limit. Your nervous system loves a dramatic entrance. A sudden drop in temperature or a sharp spike in pressure will trigger a message much faster than a steady, unchanging sensation. Your system is programmed to ignore the status quo and search for things that stand out boldly against the background.

Think of jumping into an icy pool on a hot summer day. Your system doesn't just report "cold"—it reports the massive, shocking gulf between the hot air and the freezing water. That initial plunge is a high-contrast event that completely shatters the baseline, forcing the gates open because the news is too loud to ignore.

3. The Law of Speed (The Express Wire)

This is the ultimate tie-breaker for the Sergeant of the Gate. Because safe touch and movement travel with such high velocity and in such high volume compared to danger signals, they naturally dominate the incoming communication lines. This massive speed advantage ensures that the Gatehouse news desk receives the safe data first, effectively jamming the wire and leaving the slow-moving danger signals trailing far behind.

By the time a report finally reaches the brain, it has been vetted, sorted, and prioritized by every checkpoint along the way. A properly operating Tunnel System and Gatehouse ensure that your conscious mind isn't bothered by the static of a stray sensation when there is a legitimate threat requiring your attention.

This elegant setup ensures your brain remains a high-performance command center rather than a chaotic storage unit. It handles the massive, invisible work of keeping you balanced and upright so that your conscious mind is free for higher things.

Movement as Medicine

This elegant filtering setup isn't just an automated background process; it is a system you can actively interact with. In fact, you already do it instinctively every day by using the nervous system's absolute favorite type of breaking news: movement.

Movement is the nervous system's most reliable safe signal. When you move a joint, you activate thousands of specialized sensors called proprioceptors (sensors that track your body's position in space). Because these sensors are hooked up to the lightning-fast, 250 mph express lanes we talked about earlier, moving a limb sends a massive, high-priority wave of data speeding toward the spinal cord. In a well-functioning nervous system, the gates prioritize this dynamic movement data above almost everything else, instantly pushing it to the front of the line.

This is why anxious or uncomfortable bodies rarely stay still. Pacing, shifting weight, rolling the shoulders, or even bouncing a leg under a desk are not random nervous habits. They are subconscious tactical maneuvers designed to flood the spinal gates with safe movement data, intentionally overwhelming and choking out any lingering discomfort or pain signals trailing behind in the slow lanes.

By moving, you are actively triggering the body's natural inhibitory system. Think of it as **The Law of Displacement**: your nervous system assumes that if you are physically moving or actively shaking your hand, the immediate threat is manageable. So, the Sergeant of the Gate chooses to listen to the loud headline of the movement and mute the background distress. When you burn your hand on a hot mug and shake your wrist out, the heat from the coffee didn't actually drop; the danger signal simply lost the speed competition and never got past the gates in your spine.

The Art of the Override

Up until now, we've focused on what happens at the gates themselves. But your brain uses a more sophisticated strategy. It doesn't just open and close doors. It adjusts the volume of the signals.

Sometimes it does this chemically, and sometimes it does this dynamically.

Your Internal Pharmacy

Did you know that your body has its own pharmacy? It can manufacture painkillers on demand, producing what is, in effect, a form of morphine, helping to blunt pain before it reaches full awareness. The signal is still there, but it is inhibited at the spinal cord by a release of internal chemicals.

When survival or focus demands it, your brain releases substances that bind to the same receptors targeted by morphine. Scientists have given these substances a name: endorphins.

The word comes from "endogenous morphine," meaning morphine made inside the body. Not because it is identical to morphine, but because it works on the same opioid receptors and blunts pain in a strikingly similar way.

So let's take a look at how your body uses these natural painkillers to run its own inner pharmacy.

Focus Outranks Pain

Imagine an athlete in the middle of a championship game or a parent rushing into a burning building to save a child. In these high-stakes moments, the brain realizes that survival requires absolute focus. If the brain allowed every danger signal to get through, a twisted ankle or a singed hand, the person would stop moving, and the mission would fail.

So, to prevent this, the brain releases its own flood of internal chemicals created in your internal pharmacy.

These high-grade painkillers are dispatched on orders from high command down to the spinal checkpoints, instructing the Sergeant at the Gate to manually lock down the gates and slash the intensity of the danger signals before they can even head up the tunnels toward the brain.

This is healthy prioritization at its finest. You might not even realize you've scraped your knee or bruised your shoulder until the game is over and the brain finally gives the order for the pharmacy's effects to wear off.

The Art of the Fade

But your body doesn't rely on a high-stakes chemical flood for everyday life. Most of the time, your nervous system works much more subtly. It doesn't need an emergency drug to keep the peace; it simply chooses what to listen to.

To do this, your brain is constantly sliding the faders up and down within your parietal lobe. This is the part of the brain that acts as your sensory dashboard. It is responsible for background suppression, the ability to dim the lights on unimportant data so the important things can shine. It's responsible for increasing the volume on the gentle breeze on your skin. Damping the static of your shirt against your arms or the constant pressure of your shoes. Instantly muting the entire orchestra of background data to let a single warning scream through if you step on a thumbtack.

This constant adjustment ensures that you are aware of what matters and protected from what doesn't. It is the reason you can sleep through the sound of a fan but wake up instantly when it turns off. Your parietal lobe has decided the fan is part of the wallpaper, and it's absence is a very relevant data point.

Working alongside this dashboard, your thalamus acts as the brain's executive switchboard. Unlike the gates in the spine, which only decide whether a signal may pass, the thalamus determines where it will be sent and how loudly it will arrive. Some signals are broadcast to the conscious brain at full volume. Others are simply routed to storage or dismissed entirely.

This is similar to what neuroscientists call **the cocktail party effect.** In a crowded room, you hear dozens of voices at the same intensity, but you don't consciously register most of them. This switchboard suppresses the irrelevant chatter and selectively amplifies the signal that carries personal meaning, like your name. The sound of your name isn't louder in the room; it is louder in perception because it's been prioritized. Until the thalamus forwards the message to conscious awareness, pain has not yet become a conscious experience. The signal is present, but it has not yet been interpreted.

However, the thalamus doesn't work in a vacuum. It is in constant, lightning-fast communication with the rest of the brain to determine not just what is happening, but what is about to happen.

This is the secret to the system's efficiency: the brain doesn't just respond to signals; it anticipates them. To keep your nervous system from being overwhelmed, your brain creates a pre-approved list of sensations it expects to feel based on your own movements.

This is why you can't tickle yourself. When you move your own fingers toward your ribs, your brain recognizes that it is the author of the movement, so it sends a stand-down signal to the thalamus before your fingers even touch your skin, essentially saying, "I know this person; they're with me." Because the system knows exactly who is responsible for the sensation, the gates are held shut, revealing that, as neuroscientist Karl Friston explains, the brain is essentially a prediction machine. It doesn't just wait for the world to happen to it; it anticipates the world so it can prioritize what actually matters.

That means that if a friend reaches out to do the same tickling, and your brain lacks that insider information, it can't predict the touch, so it can't pre-approve it. The gates fly open, the signal is escalated, and you burst into laughter. This is your brain successfully telling the difference between the predictable self and the unpredictable other. The thalamus has forwarded the signal, and the conscious brain has finally processed the data.

The Pianist

This predictive prioritization isn't just for survival; it is the secret to human excellence. Think of a concert pianist mid-performance. To hit every note with perfect velocity and emotion, her brain must effectively mute the sensation of the sleeves of her gown rubbing against her shoulders, the pressure of the stool beneath her, and even the minor ache in her tired forearms.

The thalamus filters out these background noises so her brain can devote 100% of its bandwidth to the music. In this state, her brain is doing something incredible; it is optimizing for beauty. This is another masterpiece of prioritization that allows our bodies to become transparent vessels for highly complex skills.

The Cold Pressor Test

While the pianist's focus is instinctive, science has proven that we can actually trigger this *mute button* on demand. To prove that the conscious brain can manually override the gates, researchers often use what is known as the Cold Pressor Test.

In this experiment, participants are asked to submerge their hands in a bucket of ice water for as long as possible. Normally, the danger signals from the freezing water reach the thalamus and scream for an immediate exit. The sensation is intense, and most people pull their hand out within seconds as the neurological alarm reaches a crescendo.

However, researchers found they could change the results without changing the water. If they gave participants a mission, such as a complex math problem to solve or a high-stakes competition to win, their tolerance skyrocketed. By shifting your brain's focus to a higher priority, the brain effectively mutes other incoming signals.

The water was still freezing. The sensors in their skin were still sending frantic danger signals, but because their conscious brain was occupied with a more *important* task, it prioritized the math over the pain. This experiment proves that your gates aren't just thermometers measuring temperature; they are active filters waiting for instructions from the top.

The Necessity of Silence

Beyond these deliberate acts of mental focus, your nervous system is working to maintain this same protective boundary every single second. We often think of silence as the simple absence of noise, but in the human body, silence is the result of perfect gatekeeping.

When your system is functioning at its peak, the Gatehouse runs like a well-commanded post. The Sergeant of the Gate stands his ground with seasoned authority, holding the endless stream of routine sensory dispatches at the threshold and ensuring that only the most relevant reports ever make it through to your conscious command. This is a masterpiece of prioritization: the Sergeant's ability to decide that the pressure of your clothing is noise to be held at the gate, while the texture of a loved one's hand is a dispatch worth waving through.

Without this active holding of the line, you could never get lost in a sunset or hold a deep conversation. You would be too busy receiving every report your body generates: the movement of your diaphragm, the constant friction of your shoes, the hum of your own pulse. Silence in your body is not the absence of signals. It is the Sergeant doing his job so well that only what matters gets through. It is the space required for a meaningful life.

By guarding who comes through the gates, your nervous system grants you the mental space to actually live in the world rather than just being a prisoner to the raw input of your own tissues.

By the time a signal finally reaches your brain, it has been vetted, sorted, and prioritized by every gate along the way. Your spine ensures that your conscious mind isn't bothered by the murmur of a stray sensation when there is a wound that requires your attention. In a healthy body, the most important work happens in the shadows, at the gates, before you ever even know there was a choice to be made.

This is the ultimate goal of the Sergeant of the Gate: to filter the commotion so effectively that you can engage with your life without being interrupted by the noise of your own internal processing. When the system is in this state of perfect prioritization, it achieves that rare, deep safety described by Kurt Vonnegut: '*Everything was beautiful and nothing hurt.*' It isn't that the world stopped sending signals; it's that the thalamus is doing its job so well that only the beauty makes the cut.

The Resilient Mind

In a healthy system, your gates are not meant to stay propped open forever. They are part of a temporary emergency response. To understand the gates, we have to accept the central blueprint of your nervous system, summarized by Lorimer Moseley's landmark observation that "pain is a protector." It is a high-level strategy designed to keep you safe while you heal, not a punishment for being injured. And like any good protector, it knows when its job is over.

Neutralizing the threat triggers a beautiful, coordinated recovery deep within your tissues. With healing comes a sweeping shift in the biological environment: inflammation cools, chemical irritants dissipate, and the local nerve endings finally stop reporting a crisis. This quiet landscape naturally chokes off the volume of danger signals dispatched into the spinal cord. At the gates, the frantic pounding slows to a gentle tap, and eventually, fades to absolute silence.

Of course, not every condition follows this exact path. Sometimes the original tissue issue remains. In those cases, the same principle still applies: the nervous system can become less protective even when the underlying condition has not completely disappeared.

However, healing isn't just about changing the tissues; it is about retraining your system to see your body differently. As philosopher Marcel Proust famously observed, the real voyage of discovery isn't about finding new landscapes, but about "having new eyes." When your nervous system stands down, it is essentially looking at the same landscape of your body, but through the eyes of safety rather than the eyes of threat.

These safe signals act as a calming influence flooding your spinal cord and brain with reports of normal, rhythmic, non-threatening activity. Their presence provides the evidence your system needs to hear: "*The crisis is over. We are back to our normal routine.*"

Standing Down

When this data floods the system, your conscious brain performs a critical piece of bookkeeping: it evaluates what you are actually doing with your body. Which means that **your brain doesn't wait to feel better before it allows you to move; it waits to see you move before it allows you to feel better.** By weighing the declining reports of danger against the overwhelming evidence of safe movement, your mind makes an executive decision to lower the alarm, stand down, and return to baseline.

With the executive order given, the gates in your spinal cord return one by one to being selective filters rather than open floodgates. Becoming less reactive and far more discerning, they stop guessing that every sensation is an incoming threat. Instead, they slip back into the quiet background work of monitoring your world without disrupting it. As the entire system recalibrates, the gates grow heavy once more, anchoring your nervous system back into the peaceful operation of daily life.

The Masterpiece of Protection

This is the true blueprint of your internal fortress. By guarding the thresholds, vetting the data, and knowing exactly when to stand down, your nervous system grants you the rare mental space required to fully live in the world rather than just constantly reacting to it. In a healthy body, the most critical work always happens in the shadows, at the gates, ensuring that you are always protected, always prioritized, and always safe.

When this system functions at its peak, it achieves a flawless balance between vigilance and freedom. It understands that a fortress is not meant to be a hiding place or an impenetrable bunker locked away from the world; it is meant to be a secure base of operations. The gates are active, dynamic filters, lowering the iron portcullis to keep real danger out, but lifting it wide to welcome in movement, connection, and joy. It is a masterpiece of biological prioritization; a design engineered entirely to filter out the relentless static of physical survival so that your conscious mind can experience the beauty of being alive.

Without this hidden foundation of safety, the things we value most in the human experience would simply slip away. Only when the system falls quiet can you look past the internal processing of your own tissues, step away from the defensive walls, and turn your gaze outward. It is this profound physical peace that lets you lose yourself in a sunset, focus on a deep conversation, or hold a loved one's hand without interruption. Far more than a survival mechanism, your nervous system beautifully curates your reality, managing the noise so you are free to step out into the sunlight and engage with your life.

5

The Captain of the Guard

How Your Brain Learns to Predict Danger

"Deep within the soul... there is a loyalty to the past that even the present cannot break."
— Carl Jung

We've already walked the inner corridors of the fortress. We've met the Sergeant of the Gate, watched him screen the endless stream of incoming dispatches, and seen how he decides what gets held at the threshold and what gets waved through to your conscious command. You understand now that the gate is not a passive opening. It's a managed post.

But the Sergeant of the Gate doesn't decide what is dangerous. He decides what gets through. The question of danger belongs to someone with a broader view and a longer memory.

Enter the Captain of the Guard

Deep within the Inner Keep, past the gatehouse and up through the winding corridors of the fortress, there is a room that never goes dark. Maps cover every wall. Dispatches arrive continuously from sentinel posts across the entire perimeter. Filed reports stretch back years, some decades, each one cataloguing the precise conditions that surrounded every past breach, every threat, every moment the fortress came under attack.

This is the Watch Room. The Watch Room is not a single chamber but a network of interconnected posts deep within the limbic system, with its command center rooted in the amygdala, the fortress's most ancient and battle-hardened threat assessment hub. And seated at its central table, cross referencing every incoming report against the archive of past incidents, is the Captain of the Guard.

He is not processing traffic. He is reading patterns and comparing them with historical records. He doesn't keep these records himself. That work belongs to the Master Librarian in the Memory Archives. But the Captain of the Guard knows her files intimately, and when a dispatch arrives that resembles a past threat, he has her records on his desk before the ink is dry. While the Sergeant of the Gate manages the threshold in the present tense, the Captain of the Guard operates across time, continuously comparing what is happening now against everything that has ever happened before. His mandate is not to manage the flow. It is to assess the threat. And his singular, ironclad command has never changed: **keep the inhabitant alive at all costs.**

He is loyal. He is tireless. And as you are about to discover, he has been on duty for a very long time.

In the previous chapters, we looked at the architecture, the wires, the gates, and the relay stations. But a fortress is more than its stone and mortar. A fortress is only as effective as the logic of the people running it. If the Sentinels are the sensors on the wall, the Captain of the Guard is the veteran officer who interprets their frantic shouts. From here forward we will simply call him your Guard, with a capital G, because that is precisely what he is: not one sentinel among many, but the historical commanding intelligence behind every protective decision your fortress makes.

The Captain at His Best

Consider what your body navigates on an ordinary day. You sip from a hot cup of coffee and your hand pulls it back a fraction of a second before the heat becomes a burn. You walk through a crowded parking lot at night and your muscles quietly tighten, your senses sharpen, and your pace adjusts, all without a single conscious instruction from you. And, by the time you reach your car, the Guard has already stood down.

This is the Captain of the Guard doing his job perfectly. He's not waiting for damage to occur before he acts. He's reading the incoming dispatches from the Sergeant of the Gate, cross-referencing them against the Master Librarian's historical records, scanning his wall maps for patterns, and issuing protective verdicts in fractions of a second. In a healthy system, those verdicts are accurate, proportionate, and temporary. The alarm sounds, the body responds, the threat passes, and the Captain stands down, and life goes on.

The Guard is the reason you survived childhood. Every skinned knee that taught you not to run on wet pavement, every near-miss that made you look both ways, every moment of instinctive recoil from something genuinely dangerous: that was the Guard writing new entries into his field manual and updating his maps. His never again policies aren't born as problems. They are born as wisdom. (We haven't talked about never again policies yet)

In a well-regulated nervous system, the Watch Room is one of the most elegant command centers imaginable. The Guard receives thousands of dispatches every hour and processes them with quiet efficiency, escalating what needs escalating, discarding what doesn't, and returning the fortress to a state of calm so reliably that you never notice he was working at all, which means his greatest successes are invisible. You only feel his presence when something genuinely warrants your attention.

That is the Guard at his best: fast, loyal, accurate, and proportionate. A protector who sounds the alarm when it matters and stands down when it doesn't.

The problem isn't a lack of protection. It's a loyalty so absolute that under sustained and unrelenting pressure, it stops distinguishing between a battlefield and an ordinary day.

But here is the problem with someone whose only metric for success is survival: He doesn't care if you're comfortable. He doesn't care if you can sit through a movie, go for a run, or pick up the groceries without flinching. To the Guard, a successful day is a day where you didn't die.

If that means keeping you locked in a dark room because he's convinced the light is a threat, he will consider that a victory.

Most people living with overprotective pain feel like their body has betrayed them. It's a deeply disorienting kind of sabotage, where the security system meant to keep you safe starts treating *you* like a prisoner. But the opposite is actually true: your system isn't failing, it's just operating in a state of permanent high alert, effectively locked into a cycle of over-protection and exhaustion from trying too hard to keep you safe.

Think of a veteran bodyguard who has been stationed in a high-threat situation for too long. He doesn't just watch for assassins; he starts seeing a threat in every stranger who reaches into their pocket for a cell phone. He hasn't lost track of reality; he's just optimized for survival, having surrendered to the exhausting safety of permanent hyper-vigilance.

Like this bodyguard, the overprotective Captain of the Guard becomes an elite specialist in your specific history, having memorized the exact scent of the air, the time of day, and the specific tilt of your spine that preceded the last time you were hurt. In his world, reaching for a grocery bag isn't a chore; it's quite possibly a high-risk maneuver. He is fiercely loyal to a version of you that was once in danger, and refuses to believe the war is over.

The Guard in the Jungle

The absolute, terrifying depth of this physiological loyalty is best captured by one of history's most extreme cases of over-training: the story of Hiroo Onoda.

In 1944, Onoda, a Japanese intelligence officer, was stationed on Lubang Island in the Philippines. His orders were simple: Hold the island at all costs and never surrender. A year later, the war ended. The atomic bombs were dropped, the treaties were signed, and the world moved on, but Onoda didn't.

For the next 29 years, he lived in the dense jungle, surviving on bananas and coconut milk and occasionally scavenging cattle from local farmers, ignoring every sign that the world had changed.

When the Philippine government dropped leaflets from planes telling him the war was over, he dismissed them as "enemy propaganda." When his own brother stood in the jungle with a megaphone and called out to him, Onoda believed it was a trick, a clever ruse by the enemy to lure him out of hiding.

Onoda wasn't acting out of madness; he was acting out of an absolute, unyielding commitment to his mission. Guided by an outdated map and long-expired orders, this elite soldier spent twenty-nine years fighting a ghost war, strictly executing the last command he ever received: never surrender.

When your Guard becomes overprotective, he is Hiroo Onoda. He's still in the jungle of your history, sharpening his bayonet and scanning the tree line for an enemy that left the island years ago.

And like Onoda, your Guard's surrender won't come from being told the war is over; it will come from the arrival of new, trustworthy evidence that overrides his historical evidence. In your brain, that isn't your doctor or your logic; it is **consistent, physical**

evidence of safety. Until the Guard receives that stand-down order through your actions, he will continue to treat the rustling of a leaf like a sniper's bullet. He isn't being stubborn; he is being a soldier.

Your Never Again Policies

A soldier in the field doesn't operate on guesswork; he follows a strict field manual. In your nervous system, this manual is made up of never again policies; protective, unyielding rules your brain adopted during past moments of overwhelm, high stress, or physical injury. Neuroscientists often refer to these deep-seated rules as learned associations, but inside the Watch Room, they function as absolute law. They are the automated scripts that instantly dictate whether a simple movement from your lower back is flagged as a normal physical sensation or an existential crisis.

These policies are stored deep within the survival circuits of the limbic system, and most specifically within a small, almond-shaped structure called the amygdala. Despite being roughly the size of a walnut, the amygdala is arguably the most powerful real estate in your entire nervous system. It is the Guard's command center, the place where threat memories are encoded, pattern recognition is processed, and protective verdicts are issued. It does not think. It does not deliberate. It acts, faster than conscious thought, on the single mandate it has always carried: keep you alive. You don't wake up in the morning and choose to enforce them. They run automatically in the background, serving as the Guard's standard operating procedures.

While everyone's history is unique, the manuals of an overprotective Guard almost always rely on the same core protocols:

1. The Prepare for the Worst Rule: Any sensory input that feels even ten percent familiar to a past injury triggers a hundred percent escalation of the internal alarm. Lacking a maybe setting, the Guard operates on a strict safety margin: he would rather force you to scream through a false alarm than risk you getting hurt in a real one.

2. The Scan for a Twinge Policy: In a healthy body, internal monitoring is a quiet, background process that leaves you entirely free to enjoy your day. But an overprotective Guard changes the protocol, bringing his spotlight into the foreground and continuously panning it across your tissues. Operating under the warped belief that a threat unseen is a threat unmanaged, he forces you to consciously feel every minor twitch. This relentless internal surveillance is the exact mechanism that converts peaceful baseline monitoring into the exhausting state of hyper-vigilance.

3. The Contextual Ban (Guilt by Association): A healthy brain naturally uses context to protect you—it memorizes the environment where a danger occurred so you can avoid it in the future. But an overprotective Captain of the Guard takes this survival superpower and applies it to everyday life. Getting injured at a desk means he blacklists the entire office environment. The smell of the morning coffee, the specific angle of the lighting, and the rhythmic sound of your keyboard are all logged as accessories to the crime, triggering a defensive pain alarm before you even pull out your chair.

4. **The Anticipatory Brace:** Whenever a movement is perceived as a threat, like standing up or getting out of a car, the overprotective Guard orders an immediate, massive lockdown of the surrounding muscles. Instead of the elegant, subconscious calculation a healthy brain uses to smoothly stabilize your joints a split-second before you shift your weight, this defensive system creates a rigid, involuntary internal splint. Tragically, this constant, protective bracing generates far more physical compression and pain than the actual movement ever would.

The problem is that once a "never again" type policy is written, the Guard won't just unlearn it after some time has passed. This is the exact moment where our third operating assumption—that overprotective pain completely reverses the order of healing—becomes an inescapable reality. Waiting for an all-clear signal before you dare to move completely misreads the situation. In fact, by staying perfectly still, you unintentionally confirm the Guard's worst fears, signaling to him that the threat is still actively lurking outside. This structural paralysis keeps his finger firmly glued to the panic button, continuously triggering the very pain you are trying to avoid.

So, the the Captain of the Guard needs a stack of new, consistent evidence, repeated experiences of safe movement, before he'll pick up his pen and cross out a rule in his manual.

But providing that evidence is a challenge because the he isn't just sitting by, waiting for you to prove him wrong. He is actively working to ensure he isn't surprised again. But before we can feed him a new stream of information, we have to reverse-engineer how he gathers his data in the first place.

How the Captain of the Guard Scans the Horizon

The Captain of the Guard, your brain's protective threat-detection system, isn't a passive observer. He is constantly scanning the horizon with high-powered telescope, looking for anything that resembles the last time the fortress was breached.

What we need to understand now is the optics of that telescope, because that is how we are going to smuggle in the new evidence he needs to see. If you try to change everything at once, you'll trip every alarm in the Keep, but if you understand what he's looking for, you can start to move in ways he doesn't immediately flag as a never-again violation.

In neuroscience, we call this associative learning. In the fortress, we call it The Patrol. The Patrol refers to the Guard's active enforcement of his policies; he is perpetually scanning the perimeter, so to speak, checking the environment against his list of known threats. He isn't just looking for physical injury or damage to the walls. He is looking for a specific Threat Signature, a toxic combination of sensation, context, and emotion. When these three things happen at once during a traumatic or painful event, the Guard fuses them together so tightly that they seemingly become inseparable. From that moment on, he treats them as a single, dangerous unit. If he sees the context (like your office desk) or feels the emotion (like deadline stress), either one, he assumes the sensation (the pain) must be right behind it, and he sounds the alarm before you've even moved a muscle. To dismantle that unit, let's look back at how they were fused together in the first place.

The Anatomy of a Trigger

Remember the first time your back went out. Maybe you were bending over to pick up a laundry basket, or maybe you were stressed about work or fearful of that sickening pop or tearing sensation you felt deep in your lower back.

If the Guard was in an overprotective state, he didn't just record, "*Watch out for heavy laundry baskets*," he generalized. And then he went about associating the act of bending, the feeling of being rushed, and even the room where it happened with the threat of catastrophe.

Now, fast forward six months. Your back is fine. But you walk into that same room, see a basket on the floor, or feel a deadline looming, and before you even reach for the handle, the Guard sees the threat signature forming. Because of that, he doesn't wait for you to bend; he sounds the alarm immediately. He tightens your spinal muscles into a protective suit of armor and floods the system with pain: reacting not to a current injury but a predicted one.

The Cello in the Water

To better understand how the Captain of the Guard fuses things together into a threat signature, we need only look at one of the most famous pieces of music in history: the two-note theme from the movie *Jaws*.

On its own, a low E followed by an F played on a cello is just two notes. It's a vibration of air; objectively harmless. But because of the way our brains learn, those two notes have been permanently fused to the image of a predator.

It plays out like this: say you are floating in the ocean and a friend who swims up behind you and whispers, "Da-dum... da-dum." You might not even pause to look for a fin or wait for an official announcement that a shark has entered the deep end, you're gonna think, "Shark!" Decades after seeing the movie and hearing that tune, your biology takes over with a cold ripple of goosebumps down your arms. Your heart rate might even kick up a notch, and your neck muscles could lock into a protective brace as you spin "nonchalantly" around. This is your Guard reacting to the soundtrack of a shark.

The sound isn't the shark, and your friend isn't a predator, but your Guard doesn't care about all that; it only cares about the pattern.

In the world of overprotective pain, your Guard has his own *Jaws* theme. For some, the music is the act of reaching for the floor. For others, it's the high-pitched whine of a dentist's drill or the specific lighting in your office.

The Guard "hears" those notes and, within milliseconds, he projects the shark (the pain) into your awareness. He doesn't wait to see if there's an actual shark. Just like the moviegoer who jumps in their seat even though they know they are sitting in a safe theater, your Guard reacts to the sound or the image of the threat, not the reality of it.

This is what makes overprotective pain so frustrating: you've got *Jaws* music playing everywhere. And ironically, you're being chased by the *idea* of a shark while you're standing in a kiddie pool, reacting to a pattern, not a problem.

The Pattern Recognition Trap

This invisible soundtrack is exactly why overprotective pain feels so profoundly erratic and unfair. Inside the Keep, it looks like madness, like the Guard has lost his mind and is blindly firing arrows at moving shadows in the woods rather than an actual invading army.

And so you don't just hurt when you lift something heavy. You feel a twinge while you're driving to the grocery store, sitting at your desk, or just trying to get comfortable on the couch.

This is a tragic case of mistaken identity in which the Guard has started to blur the lines between coincidence and catastrophe, until a minor, everyday twinge is no longer just a passing sensation, but the definitive, terrifying start of the shark theme.

Slowly, your world begins to shrink. You find yourself looking warily at a specific chair in your living room because the Guard has rebranded it as the place where the music starts. Eventually, his reach even creeps into your relationships. A tired, sharp tone of voice from your spouse or a heavy sigh from across the room is instantly translated by the Guard as an incoming attack, prompting your muscles to rigidly brace for impact before you even realize you've held your breath.

The Guard, so good at pattern recognition, has lost his ability to distinguish between a coincidence and a cause. He hears the first two notes of a song and assumes the entire orchestra is about to crash in. He sees a cloud and assumes a hurricane is coming, so he boards up the windows every time the sun goes behind a tree.

This isn't your imagination, and it isn't "all in your head" in the way people dismissively mean. It is a sophisticated, lightning-fast biological process led by an overzealous Guard trying to save you from a future that hasn't happened yet, based on a past that is already over.

Why the False Alarm is Actually a Doorway

It's easy to read about these patterns, the never-again policies, and the trigger associations, and feel like you are a prisoner in your own stronghold. If the Guard is this fast and this powerful, how do you ever stand a chance?

But here is the foundational truth you need to hold onto: **The Guard is a student of history.**

The only reason he is currently overprotecting you is that he is highly sensitive to information. He learned to be this way because he was trying to navigate a difficult season of your life. Fortunately, because he is a student of history, he is still capable of learning a new way to live.

The fact that your brain was able to create these complex associations is actually the greatest evidence that you can heal. It proves that your nervous system is plastic, it is dynamic, it is responsive, and it is capable of change. You aren't dealing with a crumbling wall that needs a new stone or a structural collapse that requires a brace; you are dealing with a brilliant, loyal protector who is simply working from an outdated manual. So, the Guard doesn't need to be replaced; he just needs you to provide him with new history.

When we move into the later chapters of this book, we aren't going to fight the Guard or even try to fire him. We are going to give him a safety briefing and show him, through consistent and gentle evidence, that the laundry basket isn't a bomb and the chair isn't a trap.

Your pain is a high-performance system that has been given the wrong instructions. And the same loyalty that makes the Guard so persistent is the same loyalty that will make him your greatest ally once he realizes you are finally safe.

The Man Who Couldn't Let Go

Most of us are taught that if something isn't working, we need to try harder. We need more control. But in the world of an overprotective brain, control is often the very thing that locks the fortress gates.

I (Sam) once worked with a man in his early thirties, let's call him Marcus, who came to me with a deeply frustrating issue. Despite being physically fit and seemingly healthy, he was struggling with a form of incontinence. Every time he finished using the bathroom, his body would leak a small amount, leaving him in a constant state of hyper-vigilance and embarrassment.

He had been through the gauntlet of medical testing. The results were always the same: no structural damage, no muscle weakness, no disease. On paper, Marcus was fine. But in the clinic, it was clear that the problem wasn't mechanical; it was a failure of timing.

You see, for your body to perform a release, whether it's emptying the bladder or relaxing a muscle, your nervous system has to hand over the keys. It has to move from a state of high-alert defense to a state of internal maintenance. But Marcus's system had been primed by years of high-level anxiety. His Guard was entrenched in a state of high alert, and to a brain that feels under siege, letting go feels like lowering the drawbridge in the middle of a raid. He was essentially trying to perform a physical release while his Guard was bracing for impact. Even though Marcus was trying to relax, the Guard was still standing at high alert, refusing to blink, fingers hovering over the alarm, his nervous system still stuck in protection mode. He wasn't interested in letting go; he was too busy scanning for the next attack. Every episode of leaking only reinforced the Guard's suspicion that the fortress wasn't safe, locking him into a vicious loop of vigilance where the very act of release is treated as a security breach.

Our intervention had nothing to do with strengthening his muscles. In fact, Marcus was already too strong; he was clenching for dear life. Instead, we worked on lowering the flags of the fortress by stimulating his parasympathetic nervous system and teaching his pelvic floor to soften, helping his Guard recognize safety again.

And because of that, the symptom didn't just improve; it went away completely. Not because he gained more control over his body but because his brain finally stopped trying to control a process that was always meant to be automatic. For Marcus, loss of control wasn't the problem; over-control was.

You Can't Just Reason Your Way Out

Your Guard speaks the language of threat and safety, not English. And, he processes that language at a speed the conscious mind cannot touch.

This lightning-fast priority was famously demonstrated in the *Snake in the Grass* experiments conducted by psychologists Dr. Vanessa LoBue and Dr. Judy DeLoache. They wanted to know if the human brain was naturally biased toward seeing threats over neutral patterns.

In their studies, participants were shown groups of small pictures on a screen. Each group contained one target image among many distractor images. The targets could be snakes or spiders, while the distractors were neutral objects like flowers, mushrooms, frogs, or caterpillars.

Participants had to locate the target as quickly as possible. When the screen was filled with pictures of flowers, and a single snake hidden among them, people spotted the snake almost immediately.

But when the screen was filled with snakes and one single picture of a flower, the search took longer. The harmless thing was harder to find than the dangerous one.

The results were a masterclass in the Guard's efficiency: across the board, the human brain identifies the threat pattern significantly faster than it identifies the safe one. Our systems are essentially pre-tuned to find the danger in the data.

LoBue and DeLoache's work proves that the Guard operates on a fast-track circuit. He isn't interested in the aesthetic details of the flower; he is scanning exclusively for the outline of a threat. This is a high-performance survival trait. The Guard would rather you jump at a thousand snake-shaped sticks than get bitten by one actual snake.

This is why you can't think your way out of a flare-up. When the Guard detects one of these patterns, he pulls the alarm before you've even had a chance to tell yourself, "*It's okay, it's just a little rustle in the leaves.*" But by the time your Council Chamber realizes there is no actual snake, your muscles have already braced, and the pain signal has already been sent. And you are living in the aftermath of a decision the Guard made in a fraction of a second.

As the renowned neuroscientist Dr. Antonio Damasio famously said: *"We are not necessarily thinking machines that feel; we are feeling machines that think."*

This is the vital, sobering truth of your current situation: you cannot reason your way out of a high-speed, biological pattern-recognition loop. When it comes to an overprotective alarm system, your logic is simply too slow for the fight.

The Watering Hole Principle

The Snake in the Grass experiments prove how quickly the Guard reacts, but that high-speed response is also backed by a meticulous library. The Guard keeps permanent records. Once an event has been marked as dangerous, that memory does not simply fade with time.

In the animal kingdom, fear is the most effective teacher. If a predator chases you at a specific watering hole, you don't need a second lesson; you remember it forever. Safety, on the other hand, is a slow, earned experience. You have to visit that exact same watering hole a hundred times without seeing a shadow before the Guard even considers crossing it off his watch list. This is precisely why casual reassurance from a doctor or a loved one rarely stops a pain flare-up. The Guard doesn't care about promises; he cares about historical proof.

The Cost of Vigilance

Running a hyper-vigilance campaign like this comes with a massive, hidden tax. Constant protection is metabolically expensive.

In a peaceful kingdom, the Guard sleeps. The gates are manned by a skeleton crew, and the fortress's wealth is spent on simply building, creating, and enjoying life. But when the Guard adopts a permanent wartime footing, the rest of the city starves. He stays on the ramparts 24/7, burning through your limited daily fuel on repeat.

This is why overprotective pain is rarely just about pain, but it is almost always accompanied by a crushing, unexplained baseline fatigue. When your Guard is constantly scanning the grass for predators, refusing to let your muscles fully release, he is draining your resources.

Eventually, this constant vigilance shows up in your life in three distinct ways:

Mental Exhaustion: Keeping the Guard on high alert is a logistical nightmare. It is the biological equivalent of a home security system that fires a full-scale air-raid siren every time a moth flutters past the porch light. Eventually, the sheer volume of false alarms becomes a form of psychological wear-and-tear. You can't think clearly, you can't rest, and you can't focus because your entire subconscious is perpetually braced for the next siren.

Emotional Fragility: When the Guard is hogging 90% of your internal bandwidth for defense, you are left with nothing to handle the friction of daily life. This is why a spilled cup of coffee, a late email, or a minor disagreement feels like a catastrophe. It isn't that you are overreacting; it is that you are being asked to catch a new emotional weight when your arms are already shaking from the load you've been carrying since sunrise.

Physical Bracing: This is the most literal drain on your body. Keeping your muscles locked down, even by just a few tiny percent, sixteen hours a day, is the physical equivalent of carrying a heavy rucksack from morning until night.

You aren't tired because you're old and worn out; you're tired because your Guard is fighting a war that ended years ago, keeping the lights on in every watchtower, just in case.

Living in this perpetual state of high alert is a logistical nightmare that your body cannot sustain. Your cells are quite literally running out of gas trying to protect you from a threat that isn't there, leaving you trapped in a body that is utterly exhausted from defending itself. But in order to step down from the watchtowers, we have to change the rules of engagement. And rewriting those rules begins by cementing your commitment to how we move forward.

So, let's take a second look at the three operating assumptions of pain recovery introduced in Chapter 2. To drop the high alert your body is living in, you have to be fully opted-in to these three assumptions. Think of this as the Guard's final briefing before we go any further. If you can accept these three things, the blueprint for dismantling this high-alert system becomes visible. If you fight them, the Guard stays in the jungle long after the war is over.

1. Pain is an interpretation, not a direct signal from tissue

First, your body detects change. Then, your brain decides what that change means. Pain is the Guard's protective verdict, assembled from sensation, memory, context, and expectation. While tissue signals contribute to that verdict, pain is not a direct damage meter generated by your tissues. That's why pain can persist long after healing or become amplified even when the underlying condition has not worsened.

2. There are two fundamentally different categories of pain

There is ***Helpful Pain***, which protects a healing injury or alerts you to the limits of an ongoing physical condition. It acts as a ***Guide***.

And there is ***Overprotective Pain***, which reflects a nervous system that has learned to treat ordinary life as dangerous. It acts as a ***Trap***.

The challenge is that these two forms of pain often overlap. A real tissue issue can recruit an overprotective alarm system, causing the Trap to speak through the same body part as the Guide. When that happens, learning to tell the difference becomes essential.

They feel identical, but they have different masters. In the chapters ahead, we are assuming that your pain has become Overprotective. It isn't a sign of a house fire (an active injury); it's a sign of a hypersensitive smoke alarm (a system-wide overreaction). One requires a fire truck; the other requires a technician to recalibrate the sensor.

3. Action Must Precede Feeling

This is the hardest pill to swallow. In normal injury, we follow a FEEL → THINK → DO approach to healing. (I FEEL pain, I THINK I'm hurt, so I don't DO anything until the tissue is healed). Put simply, we wait for the green light of feeling better before we move.

But as we've seen, overcoming overprotective pain demands that we abandon the old instinct and adopt this action-first sequence: **DO → THINK → FEEL.**

You have to show the Guard that you are safe by moving anyway, right through the middle of the false alarm. In this new world, feeling safe isn't a permission slip you wait for; it's the prize you win at the end.

This reversal works because the Guard learns through historical experience, not logic. He doesn't need a better argument; he needs better data. By taking action while the siren is blaring, you force a system error; a split second where your brain completely expects a catastrophe but experiences survival instead. You are overwriting an outdated security manual with the only thing the Guard respects: physical proof. By following this sequence, you are proving to the system that the shadow is not a wall, and you are free to step through it.

The Power of Prediction

If Chapter 3 showed us that pain isn't a simple input-output wire, this chapter has revealed what it actually is: a prediction. The Guard doesn't sit around waiting for a telephone call from your tissues telling him damage has occurred. He works more like a weather forecaster, preparing for storms before the clouds even arrive. By instantly combining past experience with present signals, he estimates the likelihood of future danger, and when that estimate climbs high enough, protection kicks in, creating real pain before any physical injury can even happen.

This shift from reporting to forecasting changes everything about how we experience our bodies. By the time a sensation reaches your awareness, the Guard has already pre-processed the data and decided what it means. Because pain is just the Guard's best prediction of future danger, he never reacts to the present moment, but is always living ahead of it, studying patterns, remembering past threats, and bracing the body before an injury can even clear customs.

This is why pain can persist even when tissues have healed. And it's why pain can become amplified even when a tissue condition remains unchanged for a very long time. The Guard isn't waiting for proof. He's acting on probability.

Neuroscientists sometimes describe perception itself as a kind of controlled hallucination: a best guess constrained by incoming evidence. You aren't feeling your body exactly as it is in real-time; you are feeling the Guard's interpretation of your body based on his current level of concern. This is why two people can have the exact same bulging disc on an MRI, but one is running a marathon while the other is bedridden. The difference isn't the disc; it's the meaning the Guard has assigned to it.

If the Guard's manual says that bending, plus stress, equals catastrophic failure, he won't wait for a message to report a tear. He'll project the sensation of pain onto your awareness as a preemptive strike, not just because he's reacting to a structural issue, but because he is reacting to the larger pattern surrounding it.

As we leave the Watch Room of Chapter 5, we hope you have a clear picture of why the brain stays stuck. It isn't because it's against you. In fact, it is brilliantly, fiercely loyal to a set of rules that once kept you alive. But when those predictions become so rigid that they no longer respond to the truth of your reality, the Fortress stops being a place of refuge. It begins to close in.

In the next chapter, we will see what happens when the Guard's vigilance becomes a total liability, and the Fortress officially becomes a Prison.

Part III

The Fortress Becomes a Prison

6

The Always-On System

When the Brain Never Powers Down

"He who has a thousand eyes to track the shadow of a wolf will never see the rising of the sun."
— Ancient Proverb

In Chapter 5, we looked at the Guard's vigilance and loyalty. We saw how he reads his manual and reacts to the slightest hint of smoke. But when fear and uncertainty take over the fortress, that loyalty takes a darker turn. The entire protection network shifts into a permanent state of siege. The delicate filters that usually quiet the background hum of your tissues are replaced by a hypersensitive wiretap. The Guard seizes total control, overrides the Council Chamber, and becomes the Warden of a fortress turned prison for your protection.

In a healthy fortress, the Guard knows exactly how to manage the main entrance. He drops the iron portcullis to keep real threats out, but he raises it easily to let life, movement, and joy come and go. He understands that a home is a secure base of operations, not a bunker to hide in forever.

But when that same protector morphs into the Warden, his relationship with the outside world warps completely. He becomes entirely addicted to surveillance, fixating on every shadow in the woods.

If you've ever watched The Walking Dead, you know the relentless tension of trying to survive a world that never stops hunting you. In the third season, the survivors hole up inside a literal prison. They choose it for the high fences and thick concrete walls, believing that if they just stay behind those barriers, they'll finally be safe.

And for a while, they are. But a prison is only as safe as the structural strength of its perimeters. In the show, the ultimate crisis hits when a massive, relentless crowd of walkers presses against the outer chain-link fences. The metal groans, the posts bend, and under the sheer weight of the pressure, the gates completely buckle and collapse.

This is precisely what happens inside your body when central sensitization takes hold—a medical term that simply means your central nervous system has become wound-up, oversensitive, and stuck with its volume knob turned all the way to maximum.

When the Warden Takes Over

When your internal Warden takes over, he becomes so obsessed with potential danger that he actively dismantles his own security protocols. He wants to monitor every single leaf rustling in the forest. To do this, he overrides those literal neurological gates in your spinal cord that we looked at in Chapter 4—the ones the Guard usually keeps closed to block out the background static of your body. Instead, he props them wide open for maximum surveillance, desperately searching for a threat.

Biologically, this is the exact moment the system breaks. By holding those spinal gates completely open, the Warden unwittingly invites the very disaster he's trying to avoid. The normal sensory updates from your body, the background noise of your joints, the friction of your muscles, the memories of old injuries are no longer filtered out and held back. For some people, those updates may include signals from a genuine medical condition. But when the Warden takes over, even legitimate signals can become amplified and interpreted through a lens of constant threat. Instead, they act just like that relentless crowd of walkers pressing against the fence. The sheer volume of data overwhelms the perimeter, swelling into a chaotic sensory horde that rushes straight through the broken gates and floods the courtyard of your mind.

When that overwhelming horde breaks through, the Warden panics. Just like the survivors in the show, when the outer fences collapse, he realizes the open courtyard is no longer safe. But instead of fighting to clear the perimeter, he orders a total retreat deeper into the complex. He pulls you away from the open air, flees the courtyard, and slams the heavy iron doors of the inner cell blocks shut. He trades your freedom for a desperate illusion of security, locking you inside the dark, reinforced concrete of the interior.

This is the central tragedy of the overprotective brain. To keep you safe from the fictional monsters of your past, the Warden turns your life into a maximum-security prison. You stop moving, you stop exploring, and you stop living, because your Guard turned Warden has convinced you that the only way to survive the horde is to stay locked in the dark. You are no longer hiding from the threat outside; you have become a captive of the very walls that were supposed to save you.

Stuck On High Alert

The reason the Warden keeps the communication gates open isn't that he's lazy or crazy; it's that he has developed a desperate addiction to constant information. He thinks that if he misses even one tiny vibration or one distant moan from the woods, the Fortress will fall. To understand why the Warden is so addicted to information, we have to look at the wiring of the Fortress itself.

Your nervous system doesn't actually have a true off-switch; instead, it relies on a delicate, shifting balance between two forces: the system that powers you up for action (the sympathetic nervous system) and the system that powers you down for rest (the parasympathetic nervous system). Think of them like a gas pedal and a brake pedal working in tandem to navigate a winding road.

In a healthy system, the Guard knows how to balance the two. When the sun goes down, and the gates are bolted, he eases off the gas of processing threats and predicting the future, presses the brake, turns off the sirens, puts down his sword, and lets the Fortress sleep. In medicine, this transition is called **downregulation**. It's the biological equivalent of the deep safety we discussed earlier; the moment where your body stops scanning for threats and starts repairing itself.

But when the Guard turns into the Warden, he loses the ability to downregulate. His foot is frozen flat on the accelerator.

In neuroscience, this perpetually vigilant state is known as **high baseline firing.** To visualize this, think of your nerves as the strings on a guitar. In a healthy body, the strings have just enough tension to play a clear note when plucked. But the Warden has reached for the tuning pegs and cranked them until the strings are stretched to their absolute limit. Now, you don't even have to touch the guitar to make a sound; the slightest breeze or a tiny vibration from a passing footstep causes the strings to howl.

Your Messengers in the tunnels are now vibrating with so much pent-up electrical energy that they are leaning forward into a permanent sprint. The smallest nudge sends them flying toward the Inner Keep with a frantic report.

But a report is only dangerous if someone decides to publish it. This is where the Warden's obsession with information turns into a frantic, 24-hour news cycle.

The 24-Hour News Cycle of the Prison

The result of your system always being on high alert is a state called hypervigilance. In the earlier days of the Fortress, the Guard's predictions were flexible; he guessed at danger but was quick to stand down when the data proved him wrong. But now that he has become the Warden, he has become a slave to his own dark forecasts. He's no longer just guessing at danger; he's actively hunting for it. And because he expects to find it, he almost always does.

To understand how this hunt completely changes your daily life, we have to revisit The Gatehouse News Desk inside the brain.

In a healthy system, the Sergeant of the Gate we met in Chapter 4 runs his desk like a world-class newsroom. He relies on his three strict biological laws—Novelty, Contrast, and Speed—to decide what gets dropped on the floor as background noise and what gets broadcast to your conscious mind. He is constantly dismissing the rowdy sensory data in the stacks, killing 99% of the boring stories (like the feel of your socks or the hum of the refrigerator) so that you can stay focused on front-page news.

But the Warden has staged a coup.

Obsessed with the original injury and terrified of being caught off-guard, the Warden bullies his way into the gatehouse. He effectively overrules the Sergeant's filter. He forces him to completely abandon the Law of Novelty and the Law of Contrast, demanding a raw, unfiltered feed instead. He no longer wants a curated front page; he wants a digital scroll of every single vibration inside the Fortress walls.

In neuroscience, this state of constant, unfiltered noise is driven by a process called **disinhibition**. Normally, the high-tower offices of the brain send soothing, chemical instructions down to the Sargeant to help him keep the rowdy data stopped at the gates. But the Warden cuts those communication lines. He revokes the shushing orders and strips the latches from the gates down below, ensuring that even the slightest vibration is enough to swing them wide open.

Under the Warden's tyrannical broadcast, the Sergeant of the Gate is forced to send everything. There is no longer any such thing as a neutral signal. The breaking news ticker at the bottom of your consciousness never stops scrolling. A minor shift in your lower back isn't just a tired muscle anymore; it's a Special Report. A slight increase in your heart rate isn't just normal exertion; it's a Nationwide Alert.

To a Warden who hasn't slept in years, every one of these minor sensations is proof of a breach. He has forced the gatekeeping Sergeant to cease doing his duty to distinguish between a tired muscle and a torn ligament, interpreting the normal, everyday noise of being alive as absolute evidence that the Fortress is under attack.

When the Warden Locks Down the Joint

This non-stop news ticker isn't just happening in your head; it's altering the very fabric of your physical body.

I (Sam) once treated a man in his forties for overprotective shoulder pain. His imaging showed that the structure of the joint was intact. As we looked closer, the shoulder issue dissolved into a larger story of a system under siege.

He wasn't just dealing with a joint; he was living in a body that had forgotten how to power down. His heart raced, his digestion was failing, and his sleep was a battlefield. He was in a state of permanent red alert. What should have been a brief surge of survival anxiety had become the background radiation of his life.

Because his alarm never stopped, the Warden reorganized his entire biology around the threat. The shoulder stayed locked because a flexible joint felt like a vulnerability the system couldn't afford.

But when we shifted focus from the muscles to the nervous system, using sensory grounding and safety-signaling breath work, the Warden finally lowered the gates, his sleep deepened, his pain receded, and even his relationship with his wife got better. Once the Warden finally stopped treating every stray signal like a member of the Walking Dead he was able to heal and the Warden was the Guard again.

The Loss of Downtime

A system that's stuck in high gear loses its most important survival tool: flexibility. In a healthy Fortress, the Guard needs cycles of safety to reset his manual and rest his eyes. But in the Prison, those cycles have vanished. When the Warden is addicted to surveillance, he starts to see rest as a security risk. To him, closing the gates feels like leaving the Fortress open to an ambush.

Because he never powers down, the alarm pathways, the roads the Messengers use to report about danger, become thick, reinforced expressways. Meanwhile, the pathways for relaxation and recovery wither from disuse.

This creates a self-perpetuating cycle where the very act of watching for the fire is what keeps the heat turned up. The more your brain scans, the more threats it predicts, and the more it predicts, the less it feels it can afford to rest. This is precisely why a moment of ease can actually trigger a flare-up; when you are trapped in an overprotective state, your brain becomes so addicted to the noise of the sirens that the sudden silence feels like a trap. Predicting that the quiet is just a lull before an ambush, the Warden sounds the alarm even louder just to be safe.

By manufacturing an alarm out of thin air, the overprotective system traps itself in a vicious, closed loop. The Warden uses his own false alarms as proof that danger is everywhere, using them to justify endless nightly patrols that ensure the Prison can never sleep.

But here is the Warden's fatal flaw: every closed loop has a tactical weak point. Because the system is fueled by that intense internal surveillance, even a brief shift away from scanning, letting your attention settle on something outside your body for even a moment, can start to reduce how much the system treats those signals as urgent.

Without this interruption, however, you end up in a state of being wired but tired; your mind racing at 100 mph processing everything as a threat, while your body is completely out of fuel, locked away in the Inner Keep. Not only are you a prisoner of your brain's fear, but your body is starting to pay the price for the Warden's endless vigilance.

The Physical Cost of High Alert

When a system stays on high alert for too long, the fortress doesn't just change its habits; it physically rewires itself. We already know the Warden commands the alarm system from the Watch Room in the amygdala, but under chronic stress, he doesn't just sit quietly; he expands his territory. Which means that, in people living with overprotective pain, this region of the brain can actually become physically larger and far more reactive. It is as if the Warden has installed dozens of new monitors and louder sirens, ensuring his is always the most commanding voice in the Fortress.

This expansion comes with a biological cost. Stanford neurobiologist Dr. Robert Sapolsky famously pointed out that the human stress response was designed for three-minute emergencies, like a zebra outrunning a lion.

The tragedy of the Prison is that the overprotective brain has kept the lion in the room for three years. He has taken a system designed for a short burst of protection and forced it to run at full speed for months on end. This leads to **Allostatic Load**: the physical wear and tear on the body that occurs when your brain refuses to let the emergency end.

This is why you can't just think your way out of overprotective pain, and why standard willpower fails. Because of this load, your biology is no longer operating on logic; it is operating on a loop of survival that bypasses the prefrontal cortex (the Council Chamber) entirely. The Warden has hijacked the radio, and he's only broadcasting alarms.

Instead, normal sensory data enters the fortress fully, piling up until the courtyard of your consciousness fills with loud, terrifying, amplified static. This is the ultimate irony of your internal prison: your pain intensifies not just because of what is happening in your tissues, but because your system has stopped sorting the everyday noise of life from actual breaking news.

The Stronghold of Inactivity

The Warden's refusal to let you leave makes perfect sense once you see the hordes of threats filling the courtyard.

Just like characters in a post-apocalyptic story retreat into the deepest, darkest cells to escape the monsters in the yard, the Warden drives you deeper into the Inner Keep to get away from the noise. In your brain, this is the **Limbic System,** the ancient, windowless stronghold designed for short-term survival, not long-term living.

The Inner Keep is the biological equivalent of your bed, your couch, or the darkened room where you hide during a flare-up. In this state, your nervous system enforces a heavy biological sanction, dropping your energy to zero the moment you try to step back out into the sun.

This solitary confinement looks like what doctors call fear-avoidance. You stop bending over to pick up a pencil because your system predicts a breach. You stop going to the grocery store because your survival brain doesn't like the idea of the lights and noise. You even stop planning for the future because the Warden has confiscated your calendar, insisting that survival in this micro-moment is the only thing that matters.

This confinement leads to a physical process called **deconditioning**, but in the Prison, it is more like learned disuse. Your muscles, joints, and nervous system are perfectly capable of movement, but the Warden has revoked your clearance. If you try to push against the bars, if you try to take a walk or sit at a desk longer than he allows, he doesn't just send a warning. He triggers a lockdown. He floods the system with pain, fatigue, or brain fog to force you back into your "safe" cell.

This life of lockdown was perfectly captured over a century ago by E.M. Forster in his story, *The Machine Stops.* Forster imagines a future where humanity lives in subterranean cells, never leaving their rooms, because a global machine provides everything they need: food, music, and communication, at the touch of a button. The protagonist, Vashti, is terrified of the outside world. She has become so accustomed to the machine's protection that the idea of physical movement or unmediated experience feels like a death sentence.

This is the state your overprotective brain wants for you, and so like Vashti, you start to believe that the only way to survive is to stay connected to your own machine (your bed, your meds, your isolation) and never venture into the unfiltered air of the courtyard.

In Forster's story, the tragedy is that the people's bodies eventually atrophy until they can no longer stand without the Machine's support. This is the ultimate goal of the overprotective brain: to make you so dependent on the safety of the Keep that you forget you were built for the sun.

The Keep was only ever meant to be a temporary bunker. Whether you're recovering from a broken bone, navigating a chronic condition, or healing from a difficult season, it was never meant to become your permanent address. By locking you inside the Limbic System, as it were, your brain has mistaken motionlessness for safety.

The Prisoner

Once you are locked away in the Inner Keep, your reality starts to shift. This is the stage famously captured in Alexandre Dumas' *The Count of Monte Cristo.* The protagonist, Edmond Dantès, is locked away in the Château d'If, a fortress-turned-prison. Over years of isolation, his world gradually shrinks until it's defined entirely by the four stone walls of his cell.

Because he is starved of the outside world, Dantès starts to find intense, obsessive meaning in the smallest details: the scratching of a termite, the dampness of the stone, or the rhythm of a dripping pipe.

This is the exact psychological shift that occurs when you are locked inside the Prison that is your own body. Because your overprotective system has restricted your life to the confines of a single room, a bed, or a couch, your mind is starved of normal outside data. With nowhere else to look, your focus turns inward. You become an expert on the internal architecture of your body, finding intense, hyper-fixated meaning in every microscopic shift, pop, or twinge.

The tragedy of this phase is that the more time you spend in lockdown, the more your brain becomes convinced that the lockdown is the only thing keeping you alive. It looks at your lack of movement and thinks, "*See? We didn't get hurt today because I kept us in the Keep.*"

Mistaking this captivity for safety, the Warden honestly believes that keeping you trapped behind the walls of your own tissues is the only thing standing between you and the walking dead in the courtyard. What your brain fails to realize is that this relentless confinement has become the greatest threat to your life. You are not under attack. You are simply a captive whose protector has forgotten that the ultimate goal was never just to survive, but to thrive

The Cost of Caregiving

To see the Inner Keep in action, look at a patient I (Sam) recently saw; a woman in her fifties with fibromyalgia, chronic back tightness, and burning upper trap pain. She was a classic people-pleaser who used to be intensely active, doing everything for everyone, but now everything she used to be able to do triggered a massive flare-up.

Because her brain mistook motionlessness for safety, any direct tissue treatment I used—massage, needling, or stretching—terrified her system, leaving her agonizingly sore for days.

Even after just five minutes on a stationary bike at zero resistance, she woke up the next morning completely sore. Of course, biologically, this is impossible; five minutes of effortless spinning doesn't release massive amounts of lactic acid that would lead to soreness. Her muscles were perfectly fine, but her overprotective brain completely misread the increased blood flow and treated it like an actual injury. Because she genuinely believed that moving was doing real damage, she stopped exercising altogether, which led to weight gain that isolated her even more.

To break this loop, we had to validate her pain without reinforcing the false alarm. Treating her fear with bed rest is the biological equivalent of giving the dog a treat for peeing on the rug. Instead, I taught her that the soreness wasn't damage, it was just static on the radio.

Once she understood that her muscles were completely safe, we could finally start retraining her brain. We didn't stop the exercise; we just changed how we approached it. The next session, we went right back to the stationary bike, but we cut the time down to just two minutes. When she was sore the next day, instead of panicking and heading straight for the couch, she reminded herself it was just a false alarm and forced herself to go for a short walk. By acknowledging the discomfort but refusing to let the fear dictate her movement, she successfully broke the lockdown cycle and slowly began reclaiming her life.

Turning Up the Volume

When your system is trapped in an overprotective lockdown, your brain loses its ability to fade out the background noise. As we saw in Chapter 4, the sensory faders get stuck at maximum volume, transforming a completely safe, two-minute bike ride into a screaming internal siren.

This constant alert state triggers a brutal physical and emotional snowball. In the clinic, we see this regularly in patients who have become severely overweight and isolated, all saying the same thing: *"I used to be a competitive athlete. My whole identity was wrapped up in what my body could do."* But a single injury can change everything.

I can't tell you how many times I've treated brilliant, athletic teenagers whose lives got completely sidelined by a sudden injury or trauma. Their brain just goes into hyper-drive to protect them, cranking up the volume so high that they have to stop playing their sport. Their world shrinks, depression and anxiety kick in, and that emotional stress gives the brain even more reasons to blast the alarms, keeping them trapped on the couch.

People can get stuck in this loop for decades. I'm working with a woman in her fifties right now who deals with obesity and constant pain. If you met her today, you'd never guess it, but she used to be an elite, competitive dancer. After high school, a few major life traumas hit, her nervous system went into total lockdown, and things just went downhill from there.

For years, doctors dismissed these patients as lazy, but modern pain science proves the opposite: the vast majority are highly driven people. They didn't choose to stop moving; their overprotective brains punished them with weeks of agony every time they tried to exercise, forcing them into total deconditioning.

And that's the real trap, because when you finally try to break this cycle and move again, your brain can panic. Psychologists call this an extinction burst: a sudden, brutal spike in pain that your brain throws at you to force you back into lockdown. It's like a toddler throwing a massive tantrum right before they finally give up. Most people quit here because they assume they're tearing something or doing real damage, but in reality, they're right on the verge of a breakthrough.

But when you stay trapped on that couch year after year, your body isn't just getting weaker, it is actively adapting to a lower state of survival. Your brain is running a highly inefficient defense system that saps your vitality every single day.

The Price of Survival

Remember back in Chapter 5 when we talked about how an overworked Guard leaves you feeling totally drained? Well, when the Warden takes over, that fatigue isn't just a temporary side effect anymore. It turns into a permanent state of biological starvation.

That's the crazy thing about this whole lockdown loop: your brain's defense system is actually working perfectly, it's just working with an intensity that is completely ruining your life. And running that constant, high-alert security system comes with two massive bills you have to pay: a total loss of physical strength, and a massive drain on your daily fuel.

1. The Loss of Strength

In the early 1990s, a team of researchers and biospherians embarked on a landmark experiment in the high desert of Oracle, Arizona, building a massive, glass-enclosed dome where life could thrive without outside threats

The whole thing was an incredible feat, but the researchers quickly ran into a really bizarre problem: the trees inside the dome were growing incredibly fast, but as soon as they got to a certain height, they would just collapse under their own weight.

It turned out the creators forgot about one major biological necessity: wind.

In the wild, when the wind pushes against a tree, it triggers a survival response. The tree actually grows tougher 'stress wood' to fight back, strengthening its core and burying its roots deeper into the ground. But by shielding these trees from the wind, the dome accidentally starved them of the exact challenge they needed to grow strong.

This is the exact toll the Warden takes on you. By completely protecting you from the wind of movement and the threat of physical activity, your brain strips away your stress wood. Trying so hard to keep you safe, it actually makes you fragile.

2. The Loss of Fuel

The second bill you have to pay is pure energy. Constant, invisible panic burns through your primary fuel—glucose and oxygen—at an exhausting rate. Spending your entire daily budget on hyper-vigilance, your brain leaves you absolutely nothing left for basic maintenance and repair. So you end up utterly depleted, forced to live way over budget while buying absolutely nothing to eat.

This leaves you in a state of biological starvation. It's not that your body lacks the raw materials it needs to heal; it's that the Warden has completely locked the pantry, refusing to divert a single ounce of energy away from his imaginary war effort to actually let you mend and recover.

Failing Math

When your brain hoards all your energy for defense like this, it doesn't just make you tired; it actively starves your higher-level abilities.

I (Sam) once worked with a fifteen-year-old, straight-A calculus student who experienced this firsthand. Out of nowhere, she suddenly started failing her math exams. At the exact same time, her right leg started giving out on her.

Though there was no physical injury, her brain was so locked in high alert that it started prioritizing protection over performance and completely congested her internal pathways, pushing aside the delicate signals needed for calculus and coordination to make room for the emergency sirens.

But once we worked together to ease that systemic pressure, her leg stabilized, and her grades bounced right back to straight A's. We didn't have to repair any physical damage; her brain just reopened the gates, regaining access to the abilities that had been trapped inside all along.

The Price of Perfect Protection

When your system stays on high alert for too long, your entire biology starts to warp under the pressure. You might think of overprotective pain as a sign that your body is failing, but the reality is much more eye-opening: your body is actually succeeding at a goal that just isn't relevant anymore. Your overprotective brain has done an incredible job of keeping you alive, but in its obsession with safety, it has accidentally stalled the very things you need to actually live.

When the Warden takes over, your brain physically changes its neural priorities. Every ounce of cellular energy and oxygen is diverted away from repair and maintenance just to fuel the sirens. And here is the real trap: your brain becomes addicted to its own surveillance. It mistakes the constant internal chaos for proof that the outside world is dangerous. It starts to interpret the quiet of rest as a security risk and peace as a vulnerability.

The result is a system that has lost all its flexibility, forcing your world to shrink. Your brain isn't trying to punish you; it is trying to preserve you. But by locking the doors and restricting your movement, it has turned your sanctuary into a cell. It has forgotten that the original mission of the Fortress was never just to survive; it was to provide a secure base so you could go out and experience the world.

The iron bars of this prison feel permanent, but they are really just built from reinforced habits of protection. At the end of the day, the Warden is still just the Guard at heart. He is a weary, loyal protector who is waiting for a signal that it is finally safe to stand down. The path to freedom doesn't require us to break down the doors or fight the Warden for control. Instead, we have to learn to speak to him in the only language he understands, the language of safety, and prove to him that the crisis is over, the gates can reopen, and it's finally safe to step back out into the world.

7

The Smudged Map

The Geography of Protection

"The map is not the territory."
— Alfred Korzybski

Close your eyes for just five seconds and focus entirely on your right thumb, specifically, the exact spot where the nail meets the skin. Can you feel the faint throb of your pulse, or the temperature of the air against it? Now, without shifting your weight, try to do the same thing with the space right between your shoulder blades.

Even though nothing is touching you, you can instantly tune into those exact coordinates. You don't have to look in a mirror to know where your limbs are; your brain has a real-time, subconscious blueprint of your entire physical self.

Scientists call this internal GPS somatosensation—your brain's 3D map of your body. Every second of your life, your tissues send a quiet little ping up to your nervous system that says, *"I am here, and this is what I feel."* When you focused on your shoulder blades just now, your brain didn't have to guess. It just checked its internal radar.

But when you are trapped in the Prison of overprotective pain, that radar goes haywire. The Warden doesn't just lock the doors; he smudges the map.

The Maps

High above the Gatehouse sits the Observation Tower, your **sensory cortex**. This is the Fortress's intelligence hub. Inside, **Cartographers** spend every waking second maintaining a massive, living map of your body.

These Cartographers don't look at the world outside the walls; they only look inward. Every parcel of your body, from the arch of your foot to the edge of your eyelid, has a corresponding plot of land on their map.

In a healthy Fortress, the Cartographers are masters of precision geography. They keep a high-definition map of your exterior and your structural frame. Because you need to move through the world, your brain needs precision geography for your fingers, toes, skin, and limbs.

On this map, your thumb is a distinct territory with a sharp border that separates it from your wrist. **When a sensor at the thumb sends a report, the Cartographers know exactly which parcel sent it.** This precision allows you to button a shirt in the dark or tell the difference between a mosquito bite and a grain of sand. This is the gift of Helpful Pain: it is localized, accurate, and tells you exactly where the trouble is.

While the Cartographers keep a master GPS map of your skin and muscles, they are, however, surprisingly bad at tracking your internal organs. To the Tower, your heart and lungs are like uncharted wilderness; they don't have clear borders or specific addresses.

This is why, when an organ sends a distress signal, the Cartographers often get cross-talk on the wires. They see an alarm coming from the deep interior and, in their confusion, they pin it to the nearest high-definition map they have, often your shoulder, your back, or your jaw. In medicine, this is called referred pain. The physical land itself may be perfectly fine, but the Cartographers have mislabeled the breach.

As your Fortress shifts into a Prison, this precision geography fails everywhere. The once-clear borders of your body's map simply dissolve into a smudge. Places that used to have sharp, distinct boundaries, like your lower back, your hip, or your shoulder, suddenly bleed into one another right on the Cartographers' desks. Once that map smudges, the Tower loses its nuance, unable to tell the difference between a gentle stretch and a genuine structural crisis, the Cartographers panic. So, they pull the master lever and blanket the entire territory in a loud, blinding roar of pain.

The Use It or Lose It Policy

This total breakdown happens because the Cartographers' maps are not carved in granite. Unlike the stone walls of the Fortress, they are drawn in pencil.

In the world of brain science, this is just how neuroplasticity works. Those maps in the Observation Tower are living documents, and they need a constant stream of fresh, interesting data to stay accurate. The Cartographers follow a rigid "use it or lose it" policy: if you stop moving a part of your body, that patch of land stops sending clear signals. And when a territory goes quiet, or when it sends nothing but a monotonous, non-stop roar of alarm, the lines on the map start to drift.

But movement and everyday sensations are the pencil sharpener we need. Every single time you bend a joint, stretch a muscle, or feel a new texture, you are tracing over the map, keeping the borders dark, the geography sharp, and the Cartographers happy.

Unfortunately, when we're in pain, we tend to stop moving in order to protect ourselves. But when movement stops, your brain stops receiving the varied signals it uses to maintain an accurate body map. Without that varied stream of signals, your brain's cortical representation of that body part starts to degrade. What was once a sharply defined, high-resolution region in the sensory cortex is replaced by a messy, blurry border based entirely on your brain's defensive hyper-vigilance.

The Warden's Raw Feed Problem

Used to quiet, orderly reports, the Cartographers suddenly find themselves drowning in noise. As the Warden takes over, he fundamentally changes the rules of intelligence. No longer interested in a calm, curated front page, instead, he demands the raw, unfiltered digital feed of every single vibration, twitch, and temperature shift inside the Fortress. And this constant flood of panic data completely sabotages the accuracy of the master map.

In pure biological terms, this constant state of hyper-vigilance floods your nervous system with stress chemicals, creating a massive volume of overwhelming sensory static in the brain.

In the words of neuroscientist Adriaan Louw, your neurons are suddenly trapped in an endless, emergency "pain meeting," the Warden pulling the entire cartography staff away from their drafting tables and forcing them into the conference room to argue over the crisis. But when everyone is stuck in a defensive huddle, nobody is left at the front desk to answer the routine phone calls.

Now, because your neural bandwidth is entirely consumed by this meeting, other routine operations are abruptly canceled. This is why, under trauma or severe chronic stress, sudden physical pain shows up: a leg unexpectedly gives out, blood pressure spikes, or your working memory goes blank because the processing power required to hold those functions steady has been conscripted by the Warden.

Back in the Tower, the meeting drags on. Desperate to get something down on paper, the Cartographers start using thick markers just to keep pace with the alarms. When the lines become thick enough, they start to touch, and that is where the geography of your body starts to disappear.

The Smudging

In the medical world, this ink bleed has a clinical name: **Cortical Smudging.** It might sound like a metaphor, but it's a physical change scientists can actually see on functional brain scans. In a healthy system, the areas of your brain representing different body parts look sharp, distinct, and orderly. But in someone living in the prison of overprotective pain, those neat boundaries melt. The territories physically overlap.

The smudge is the biological signature of an overprotective brain. It shows that the nervous system is playing a major role in the experience of pain, regardless of whether a tissue issue is present. The land may or may not have changed, but the GPS coordinates the brain uses to find it have become scrambled.

Friendly Fire

When your brain's body map becomes smudged like this, your nervous system starts to misinterpret incoming signals.

And without clear boundaries between body regions, your brain loses some of its ability to sort sensory information accurately. Signals that originate in one place can spill into neighboring regions of the sensory cortex.

This triggers a kind of neurological friendly fire where a routine signal from otherwise healthy tissue accidentally lands inside a region the brain already associates with danger.

The Cartographers, unable to tell the difference anymore, treat the entire area as part of the same emergency.

The Ghost Breach

When the brain loses the clear borders on its internal map, your nervous system loses something just as critical: the ability to accurately locate the threat. Without a clear map showing where the danger begins and ends, your body can't mount a precise defense.

So your brain does what any security system is programmed to do when certainty disappears: it escalates. If it can't identify the exact location of the threat, it has to assume the danger could be anywhere within the territory.

That assumption produces what we call a Ghost Breach.

In a Ghost Breach, your subconscious defense system preemptively treats completely healthy tissue as if it were already compromised. This is the exact reason your pain feels like it is spreading: the injury hasn't moved, but the brain's map of danger has.

In a healthy state, your brain's protective threat-response is precise and efficient, like a highly targeted laser. But once your neural map loses its clear borders, your nervous system switches to a carpet-bomber approach, sending distress signals to an entire region to blanket the area with protective alarms. Suddenly, profound stiffness and aching start appearing in places that weren't even part of the original injury, simply because your muscles are being conscripted into stabilization. The result is your body spending its vast metabolic resources to fight a war against a ghost.

Sensory Fog

Living in a state of hyper-vigilance can create some unexpected biological byproducts. When your brain shifts into permanent overprotection, whether through overprotective pain or high-voltage anxiety, it reallocates its processing power, shifting resources away from precision and toward surveillance.

In the medical world, this is often referred to as **cortical reorganization.** But inside the Prison, we call it **Sensory Fog**. It is a collection of strange, non-painful glitches that make you feel like a stranger in your own skin.

Maintaining a high-definition map of your limbs is incredibly expensive. It requires a massive amount of bandwidth to process the constant stream of data coming from your nerves, and your overprotective Warden can no longer afford that luxury. To save power, he drops the resolution of your internal map down to a low-res blueprint.

When your internal map loses its resolution, your brain can no longer run your body on autopilot. It is forced to switch to a clunky manual override, trying to verify every single movement, signal, and heartbeat in real-time.

This manual override doesn't just cause pain, it creates a cascade of strange, frustrating, and non-painful neurological glitches that can make you feel like an absolute stranger in your own skin. To help you understand what is happening inside your own system, let's look at the five ways the Warden's low-res map breaks your daily life:

- **The Digital Trace & The Klutz Glitch:** Why your brain miscalculates your physical coordinates, making you drop objects and bump into doorways.

- **The Ghost Sting & Your Own Personal Static:** Why blurry folders in the brain's filing cabinet translate routine touch into burning pain and constant buzzing.

- **The Stumble in the Dark:** Why your muscles act like blind actors, navigating toward targets that don't actually exist in the physical world.

- **The Sitting Paradox:** Why a simple kitchen chair can feel like a high-wire act that burns through a whole day's worth of energy.

- **The Energy Blackout & Focus Drain:** Why the Warden blows your biological fuses, shutting down your memory, focus, and stamina to keep his security lights on.

Let's see how the first glitch takes down your physical coordination.

The Digital Trace

We already know that your brain is an active prediction machine, that it calculates danger and constructs pain based on what it expects to happen next. But this predictive power isn't just used for security; it's also the secret engine behind how you move through the physical world.

Every movement you make leaves a digital trace in your nervous system, a recorded prediction of how that movement should feel, where your limbs should land, and what the world should look like when they get there. When those traces become corrupted, the glitches follow.

When you reach for a cup of coffee, your brain doesn't wait for your fingers to touch the ceramic to know where they are. Instead, it runs a high-speed simulation, which neuroscientists call a forward model, that builds the movement coordinates a split second before your hand ever leaves your side. Your body then follows that pre-built trajectory.

This idea came to life in 1986 in an episode of the Twilight Zone called *A Matter of Minutes*. In the episode, a couple accidentally slips into the future and discovers that time is being assembled by a crew of workers who are building the scenery of the next minute. When something is missing or out of place, it's because the construction crew made a mistake. So, if the crew forgets to put your keys on the counter, the keys just aren't there when you walk into the room.

Your brain's predictive crew operates the exact same way, constantly constructing the next room of movement before your limbs arrive in it.

But inside the Sensory Fog, the construction crew is working off a low-resolution, smudged blueprint. The crew is still building the next room as fast as they can, but their measurements are completely warped. The physical movement of your arm might be perfectly executed, but the crew has built the coffee cup's landing zone three inches to the left of where it sits in reality.

When the brain's predictions land on the wrong coordinates, your daily life begins to glitch.

The Klutz Glitch

When your brain drops the resolution of your internal map to save power, the very first casualty is your physical coordination. This smudged map is the exact reason so many people trapped in the Sensory Fog suffer from a brutal, frustrating background clumsiness.

I (Hayley) am such a klutz that it must be some kind of cruel joke where inanimate objects are out to get me. If you were to hand me anything without positively recognizing that I have it, it will most certainly drop to the floor. Every time I reach for something in the cupboard without stopping to think, my hand doesn't grab it. It slaps it, sending it tumbling further and further out of reach with each failed attempt.

For a long time, my arms were permanently bruised from hitting a doorway at least once a day. I once went to sit down in my car and missed the seat. I literally fell onto the ground.

For years, I thought I was just cursed. But then I learned the truth: my brain's smudged map had led the construction crew to prepare the landing point for my body a few inches away from where reality actually was.

In neuroscience, this is called a prediction error, wherein the brain's internal model of the body makes a small mistake about where a limb will land in space. When my hand or my body moved, it moved exactly where the brain prepared the space for it to go—bang.

I didn't miss the target. I perfectly filled the space my brain predicted. The problem was that the prediction was placed in the wrong location. The movement felt correct to my nerves, but the world didn't line up with the brain's expectation.

The Phantom Sting

For just a minute, imagine your brain's sensory map like a massive filing cabinet. In a healthy state, every single body part has its own crisp, cleanly labeled folder. When a fly lands on your left elbow, the brain instantly pulls the "left elbow" folder, reads the data, and knows exactly what is happening.

But inside the Prison, it's as if a bottle of dark ink has leaked inside the drawer. The labels have smeared together. The elbow folder is now stuck to the forearm folder, and the ink from old pain has bled directly into the folder for light touch.

I (Hayley) have a close friend who frequently experiences what we call a Phantom Sting. Without any warning, she will suddenly feel like her legs are being attacked by an army of angry ants.

In reality, the Warden has just gone to pull a folder from her cabinet and found a total mess. So when he receives a tiny, routine signal from the lower body (maybe just the gentle brush of her leggings) the smeared "soft touch" and "threat" folders make it impossible for him to tell them apart.

And because the system is biased toward safety, the Warden doesn't guess it's just fabric; he guesses it's an attack, translating that blurry, misfiled data into a very real sting. And believe it or not, he can even send signals back down to the skin to increase blood flow, producing actual redness or hives where the "ants" were felt. There are no bugs, but there is a very real biological alarm being triggered by a Warden trying to read a filing cabinet where the ink has run.

The Stumble in the Dark

Even in a fully lit room, your muscles are operating in the dark. They cannot see the rug, the floor, or the chair. They navigate entirely by internal map, and when that map is smudged, the lights don't matter.

This clerical error doesn't just stay in the filing cabinet; it dictates exactly how you move.

Your muscles are essentially blind actors. They take their orders exclusively from the proprioceptive map—the internal GPS inside your brain that tracks where your limbs are in space. This creates a high-stakes sensory mismatch.

Sure, your eyes see the rug perfectly, and they can send a clear message: "The rug is exactly four inches in front of us. Lift your foot." But the Warden is looking at a smudged map that says your foot is already two inches to the left of its actual physical position.

In a healthy state, your brain resolves this conflict instantly because it trusts the eyes and updates the map. But in the Prison, the Warden is so overwhelmed, and the map is so out of whack that he stops trusting the visual input entirely. He defaults strictly to the internal coordinates.

The result is a sudden stumble caused entirely by ghost coordinates. Your blind muscles perfectly navigated to the exact target your brain prepared; it's just that the target didn't actually exist in the physical world.

The Energy Blackout

All of these glitches lead to one inevitable place: a forced system shutdown. But the blackout itself is only the final consequence. The real story begins with the massive internal power leak that sets it in motion.

In a famous 1999 experiment at Harvard, researchers asked participants to watch a video of people passing a basketball and count exactly how many times the players in white shirts passed the ball.

Midway through the video, a person in a full gorilla suit walks into the center of the court, thumps their chest, and walks off.

Half of the people watching didn't even see the gorilla because they were so intensely focused on the task of counting passes, their brains just deleted the gorilla from their conscious awareness to save processing power.

In the Prison, your pain is the basketball game.

Your Warden is so hyper-focused on counting every "pass" of pain, every "Static" buzz, and every "Stumble" that he has no processing power left for anything else. This is the **Power Leak.** It's why you can look right at your car keys and not "see" them, or listen to your spouse talk and not "hear" the words.

In a healthy state, your brain handles movement and sensation in the background; it's a low-energy, automatic process. But when the data in the filing cabinet is unreliable, the brain switches to a manual override in which it can no longer let your body just move. It has to manually verify every single signal, coordinate, and sensory input in real-time.

This creates a massive power leak. You're essentially trying to fly a 747 by hand-cranking the engines like a Model-T Ford. Every step you take and every sensation you process, therefore, comes with a massive energy interest rate. You aren't just moving your legs; you are forcing your brain to recalculate your existence with every stride.

It's like knowing how to type forty words per minute but failing as you start to pay attention to what your fingers are really doing. The second you try to find the keys consciously, you stumble. In the Prison, your Warden is trying to type your entire day, every step, every reach, every breath, by looking at the keys. No wonder the system is overheating.

This relentless mental effort is why you feel wiped out after a simple walk or a trip to the supermarket. You'll say, "I only walked for ten minutes; why do I need a nap?" It wasn't the physical effort of walking that exhausted you; it was the mental effort of the Warden trying to navigate a smudged map.

By the time you reach the checkout line, your brain has reached its computation limit. So, to prevent a total system crash, the leak finally triggers a forced Energy Blackout.

The brain pulls the master breaker and suddenly shuts down non-essential processes, like your focus, your mood, and your physical stamina. Your crushing fatigue is a forced system shutdown. It is your brain's way of pulling the lever because it has literally run out of juice to keep the map and the muscles in sync.

Your Own Personal Static (Paresthesia)

This computational overload doesn't just drain your energy battery; it also completely breaks your internal soundproofing.

In Chapter 4, we looked at how "the fade" naturally filters out the noise of your own body. We said that, in a healthy state, your brain mutes the constant pulse of things like your blood and the brush of your clothes so you can focus on the world.

Inside the Prison, however, the Warden permanently disables the fade. In the medical world, this is called central sensitization.

Disabling this natural volume dial forces your brain to process every single micro-signal from your nerves at 100% volume. This is why nearly one in three people in persistent distress experiences a persistent, frustrating buzzing, tingling, or fizzing sensation under their skin. Their brain has lost its ability to mute its own electrical background noise. What you are hearing is not necessarily damage; it is often the raw, unfiltered hum of your own nervous system.

The Sitting Paradox

The brutal interest rate of this manual override is also the secret behind one of the most baffling, invisible symptoms of the Prison: the inability to do something as simple as sit up in a chair.

I (Hayley) have lived with this computational power leak for most of my life. For years, doctors labeled it as chronic fatigue, fibromyalgia, or unexplained weakness. All I knew was that I just didn't have the stamina of other people my age. At my worst, the fatigue was so crushing that I spent an entire year barely able to leave my house.

Growing up, I was completely unable to relax unless I was completely lying down. While most people can relax by simply sitting in a chair, to me, sitting still felt like intense, exhausting physical labor.

I once went to a friend's house where they didn't have a couch; she explained that her family just "sat around the table together" to talk and relax. To her, that was rest. To me, that was a prison sentence. I couldn't understand how anyone could possibly "rest" while sitting up.

For a long time, I felt weak or just lazy because I couldn't handle a simple kitchen chair. But now I understand the physiological truth: for my friend, sitting was a low-power background program running effortlessly on autopilot. But because my internal map was so smudged, my Warden didn't trust my postural kickstand. He was treating a simple chair like a high-wire act, manually micro-managing every tiny muscle in my back, neck, and core just to keep me from plummeting to the ground. My brain was burning through a day's worth of mental bandwidth and CPU power just to keep my head over my shoulders.

Lying down was the only way to let the Warden stop calculating. When gravity was finally removed from the equation, the Observation Tower could finally close the postural program, turn off the manual override, and rest.

The Focus Drain

This relentless energy theft doesn't just exhaust your muscles; it also actively drains your personality, your patience, and your intellect.

In a telling and famous psychological experiment conducted at Case Western Reserve University, researchers put two groups of people in a room that smelled like freshly baked chocolate chip cookies. One group was allowed to eat the cookies; the other was forced to eat raw radishes while staring longingly at the cookie tray.

Afterward, both groups were given an intentionally unsolvable geometry puzzle to solve. The cookie group worked on the puzzle for nearly twenty minutes with patience and humor. The radish group? They gave up in less than eight minutes. They were irritable, frustrated, and snappy.

Why? Because willpower, focus, and emotional regulation pull from the exact same battery as physical survival. The Radish Group wasn't inherently meaner than the other group; they had simply spent all their personality credits on the agonizing effort of resisting those cookies. This shows that while the power leak hits your muscles, the focus drain hits your very sense of self.

The Electrical Grid of the Mind

Think of your brain like a house with a limited electrical grid. In a healthy state, there is plenty of power to keep all the lights on at once:

The Kitchen is bright and processing your digestion.

The Living Room is lit up and managing fluid, automatic movement.

The Library has pristine task lighting for sharp thinking and memory.

But in the Prison, the Warden believes there is a security breach in the basement; your pain and your smudged map. To fix it, he plugs in dozens of massive, high-voltage industrial floodlights and aims them at that one spot. These floodlights represent the constant monitoring and manual override we've discussed.

Because those security floodlights are hogging nearly all the electricity from your power source, the Warden has to brown out the rest of the building. This intentional brownout is what we call brain fog.

It might feel like you are losing your mind, but that is only because the Warden has decided that survival (monitoring the smudge) is more important than enrichment (remembering where you put your keys or following a plot twist). This is the cost of living in a Fortress where the Library has been closed until the Warden decides the emergency in the basement is over.

Why the Glitch Matters

Understanding the sensory fog and the relentless power leak is the only way to make sense of the absolute nonsense of overprotective distress. The Prison is not just a place where you feel pain; it is a place where your very relationship with reality has been distorted. When you miss the car seat, when your limbs feel like lead, or when the words on a page begin to blur, it is easy to believe that your body is failing or that your mind is slipping away. It is easy to feel like a stranger in your own skin.

But these glitches are not signs of permanent damage. They are the tactical maneuvers of a nervous system that has become obsessed with a single, impossible goal: total certainty.

In a healthy body, your brain allows for a margin of error. It trusts the digital trace and lets you move through the world on autopilot. Your subconscious wiring understands that a minor smudge on the map isn't an emergency; it's just being flexible in life. But in an overprotective pain loop, your threat-detection system has lost its nerve. It has traded precision for protection. Your brain would rather you be exhausted and clumsy in a safe zone than agile and alert in a zone it can't perfectly see.

This is the central tragedy of the overprotective brain: in a desperate effort to keep you safe, your central nervous system is willing to completely bankrupt your daily energy resources. It will pull the power from the brain's analytical centers, shut down the corridors of focus, and charge you a massive energy interest rate for every single move you make, all to keep those high-voltage defensive floodlights burning in the basement.

The sensory fog is the smoke from those fires. The energy blackout is the cost of the fuel. But even when the underlying tissues are stable, or when the internal blueprint has become blurry, we still have to ask a deeper question: What is keeping your subconscious defense system so utterly terrified? If the threat no longer matches the level of alarm, why does your body continue to act like the walls are falling down?

That answer lies beyond the physical hardware of the body and the digital software of the map. It lies in the dark stories the mind tells itself, and in how a simple, silent "what if?" can act like gasoline on a fire that was supposed to have burned out years ago.

In the next chapter, we will step inside The Catastrophization Cycle to explore how fear becomes the ultimate architect of the Prison, slowly turning a blurry map into a permanent cage.

8

The Catastrophization Cycle

How Fear Fuels the Prison

"Fear is a phoenix. You can watch it burn a thousand times, and still it will rise again from its own ashes."

— Leigh Bardugo

In 1995, a twenty-nine-year-old construction worker arrived at the emergency department of a hospital in the United Kingdom in a state of sheer, unadulterated agony. While working on a job site, he had jumped down from a platform and landed directly onto a six-inch steel nail.

The sight was enough to make the nurses wince: the massive nail had pierced clean through the center of his heavy, steel-toed leather boot. The man was in such distress that he couldn't even be examined; the slightest movement of his foot or even a vibration on the floor near his stretcher caused him to howl in pain. To get him through the initial evaluation, the medical team had to sedate him with powerful intravenous painkillers.

Once he was stable, the surgeons carefully started to cut away the leather of the boot to assess the damage. They expected to find a mangled foot, shattered bone, and significant blood loss.

Instead, they found a miracle. As the boot came away, the surgical team realized the nail had passed perfectly between the man's toes. There wasn't a drop of blood. There wasn't even a scratch on his skin. Physically, the man was entirely unharmed.

This case, published in the British Medical Journal, remains one of the most famous examples of a biological process called **Threat Appraisal.** His brain didn't wait for a signal from his foot to tell it how much to hurt; it simply saw the six-inch spike, recognized the context of a dangerous construction site, and pre-ordered a blinding ten-out-of-ten agony to force him to stop moving immediately. The threat was a complete illusion, but the torment was entirely real, proof that pain reflects the brain's assessment of danger, not just the state of the tissues.

When faced with uncertainty, your mind will always choose an agonizing false alarm over a fatal mistake. It would rather torture you by accident than let you get hurt by omission. This is the heart of the catastrophization cycle's survival-at-all-costs-zero-risk policy.

Prison Lore

But your brain cannot protect you without a backstory. When that construction worker looked down at the nail in his boot, his nervous system instantly activated a massive, internal narrative, something we call prison lore.

Every great fictional world runs on lore, whether it's Star Wars or Elden Ring. In these worlds, the plot is what is happening on the screen right now. But the lore is the thousands of years of history that happened before you even turned on the game or sat down in the theater.

Lore is the essential answer to the question of why their world is the way it is. Lore explains why a specific forest is feared by everyone in the village, why two groups of people have been at war for centuries, or why a specific sword is considered cursed. Lore gives context to every action. Without lore, a dragon is just a giant lizard; with lore, that dragon is the ancient, vengeful guardian of a fallen kingdom.

In these stories, there is usually an origin event; a Great War or a terrible prophecy. And once that event happens, the world changes its rules to make sure it never happens again. The people build massive walls, they stop trusting outsiders, and they live in a state of constant readiness. And generations later, the people are still hiding behind those same walls, having forgotten the war itself, but not the Lore, which dictates their lives and keeps them in a state of fear.

Not surprisingly, your brain has its own version of this.

Your origin event might have been a car accident, a sports injury, or a period of intense emotional stress. And in response, your brain rewrote the rules of your body to make sure you never got hurt like that again, building walls of tension and setting up no-go zones for certain movements for your protection.

Fortunately, in a healthy system, the Fortress's **internal library of past experiences** and **what-if scenarios** is just a reference section. If you feel a twinge in your back, your brain might briefly recall a story about a time you overdid it at the gym, but it quickly checks the current data, sees no evidence of actual catastrophic damage, and lets the story fade into the background. In other words, the lore doesn't change the reality of the moment.

But in a state of overprotective pain, your survival brain stops checking reality and starts living inside Prison lore.

Rather than comparing the story to your body, your brain begins to build your body out of the story. That means that if your internal lore is filled with warnings about being prone to migraines or living with permanent damage, your brain, in a truly defensive maneuver, starts responding more to the forecast than the evidence.

For over ten years, I (Hayley) lived inside an embarrassingly bizarre piece of personal lore: I was completely convinced that wearing jewelry triggered my headaches. In my mind's script, the slight pressure of earrings or the weight of a necklace against my skin was a direct line to a debilitating flare-up. So, I stopped wearing them entirely.

For a decade, my nervous system operated under an absolute law that jewelry was dangerous. The moment I put on a pair of earrings, my brain wouldn't wait for an actual physiological trigger; it just bypassed physical reality, consulted the ancient lore, and started manufacturing a headache to force me to take them off.

But I'm happy to report that now, I wear jewelry every single day. But getting here took time. I had to start in tiny doses, putting on a necklace for just a few minutes to prove to my brain that nothing bad would happen. It meant leaning into the discomfort and doing it even when I didn't feel like it. Piece by piece, I rewrote the lore until the loop finally broke.

The Simulation Trap

We build these painful bodily realities through what psychologists call catastrophizing. It's tempting to think of this as just a bad habit of worrying too much, but inside an overprotective nervous system, a catastrophic thought isn't passive; it is a High-Intensity Threat Rehearsal.

Overprotective pain is often the result of the rehearsals that hijack your Threat Appraisal system. In this rehearsal, you go over the disaster so many times that your brain's appraisal filter becomes hypersensitive to that particular threat. In the case of the construction worker, his brain didn't even wait for the nail to pierce the skin; it just started sounding the alarm because he'd been practicing for just that occasion.

Every time you imagine the worst-case scenario, you aren't just overthinking; you are issuing a command to the Warden to run a full-scale emergency drill. And if you run the disaster script in your head a thousand times, your brain logs that as a thousand separate emergencies.

The False Warden

This creates a structural problem because your brain's threat system is not calibrated by truth; it's calibrated by frequency.

Modern neuroscience has validated this prediction process through a **principle known as Hebb's Law, which states that** "neurons that fire together, wire together." Meaning that when your brain repeatedly experiences a specific sensory input (like lifting a heavy box or hearing a loud noise) at the same time it experiences stress or pain, those two groups of neurons fire simultaneously. Then, to make future communication faster, your brain builds a high-speed neural shortcut between them.

Because of Hebb's Law, each catastrophic loop strengthens the predictive pathways in your cortex. Which means you are effectively training your brain to operate on projection instead of perception. Which means that you stop asking, "*What is happening right now?*" and your default becomes, "*What is the worst thing that could happen, and how do I prevent it immediately?*" This is where the Guard turned Warden takes over.

You might feel like you are making a completely logical, cautious decision to stay on the couch or avoid a certain movement. But you aren't. You are just executing a preloaded emergency script developed by your own rehearsal.

Preparation vs. Conditioning

If you are living with prison lore, your mind is almost certainly running these worst-case scenarios on a loop. And honestly? It makes complete sense why you do it.

When your body feels volatile or unpredictable, worrying doesn't feel like a mistake—it feels like basic survival. It's like knowing there is a tiger hiding in the brush right around the corner, just waiting to pounce. Subconsciously, we tell ourselves that if we can just stay hyper-focused on that threat, we won't be blindsided when it jumps out. We think that tracking the monster's every potential move is the only way to brace for the impact. It feels like preparation.

But there is a hidden hitch in how the brain processes that safety net.

Biologically, your nervous system would rather prepare for a tiger that never arrives than be caught off guard by one that does. So every rehearsal teaches your brain to start acting as though the tiger is already in the room. Which means that every time you mentally brace for the catastrophe, you're training your brain to hunt for danger around every corner.

The irony of it all is that this doesn't actually prepare you for anything. Instead, the constant rehearsal just physically lowers your threshold for pain. It rigs your internal sensors so tight that the mere rustle of a leaf is treated like a lethal attack, and things that used to be a little uncertain now read as a definitive threat. And things that were once just uncomfortable now feel completely unlivable.

Tragically, you haven't built a defense against the tiger; you've just trained your brain to start tearing you apart before the monster even arrives.

Enforcing the Lore

Once your brain is fully convinced that the predator is lurking in the brush, passivity flies out the window. Defending you from an imaginary threat requires a radical, top-to-bottom overhaul of how your internal system processes reality—a total rewriting of its daily operations to enforce the survival script.

In a clinical setting, this systemic overhaul is what doctors try to measure using the **Pain Catastrophizing Scale** (PCS). Why do they care? Because decades of data show that a high score on this scale is the single greatest predictor of whether an injury will turn into lifelong overprotective pain. It tells a doctor that the problem is no longer explained by the structural issue alone; the brain's alarm system has become part of the story.

On a doctor's clipboard, it looks like a psychological profile, but inside the prison of overprotective pain, it's the exact three-part tactical method the Warden uses to keep your entire system under his thumb.

Magnification

Magnification is what happens when your brain turns your attention into a stethoscope.

This process directly sabotages the "art of the fade" we talked about in Chapter 4; the biological background suppression that dims routine bodily data so you can have a life without constantly monitoring your body. But the moment you become convinced that a specific part of your body is broken or unstable, your system stops fading and turns on active monitoring, pressing that stethoscope hard against that single spot.

Think about a minor knee injury. It might stay sore for a few weeks (nothing catastrophic) but if your nervous system goes on the defensive in a frantic bid to protect you, your brain deploys intense, hyper-focused surveillance to that spot. It opens up a live audio channel to that single joint, overriding the fade and locking your conscious mind into a state of perpetual listening.

Once that's done, pain comes at you out of nowhere throughout the day, not just because of the state of the knee itself, but because your nervous system has turned up the volume on that location. In this instance, your tissue isn't failing; your system is just listening too hard. Helpful Pain points to a problem. Magnification turns that problem into the center of your attention.

Rumination

Once the volume is turned up, your system enters a state of rumination. If Magnification is the act of opening a live microphone to your injury, Rumination is turning your mind into a chaotic open mic night in which your system completely loses its quality control, handing the stage to your deepest anxieties and putting that raw audio on an obsessive tape loop; leaving the exact same horror story of how you were wounded playing in your head twenty-four hours a day.

This looping is driven by a specific neural circuit known as the **Default Mode Network** (DMN). In a healthy Fortress, this network acts like your brain's passive background mode. Designed to switch on only when your mind is idling, the DMN allows you to daydream, process your day, and mentally recover.

But when your internal lore is dark, quiet time is effectively hijacked. So that the moment you try to relax, the DMN activates, automatically handing the microphone over to those looping thoughts.

The tragic irony of Rumination is that you end up trapped on a down-escalator, forced to walk up it forever, only to stay in the exact same place. Your body is desperate to rest, but your nervous system is stuck in an exhausting, involuntary climb.

Driven by the primal conviction that stepping off means letting a catastrophe catch up, your relentless mental movement never stops. And outrunning a ghost becomes your brain's sole, exhausting directive.

Helplessness

Not surprisingly, sustaining this level of hyper-focused surveillance and non-stop looping eventually blows a fuse, and forces your nervous system into the full stop of Helplessness.

In the wild, when an animal is caught in a predator's jaws and can't fight or flee, its nervous system triggers the freeze state. It plays dead and completely surrenders because fighting back will only waste energy and cause more damage.

In overprotective pain, helplessness is the freeze of Fight/Flight/or Freeze. Your brain looks at the dark lore, decides that fighting the pain is a losing battle, and orders a total shutdown. Shutting off the pharmacy, it tries to conserve energy for a catastrophe it thinks you can't prevent.

The ultimate tragedy is that your brain thinks this surrender is protecting you, when it's actually leaving you completely exposed to more pain.

The Backdoor of The Brain (Signs and Superstitions)

If standing orders are how the Warden enforces the lore, then triggers are the scouts that tell him when to call in the troops. Most people think pain starts when they move, but for a brain steeped in lore, it mostly starts with an association, and the pathway runs through the back door of the Fortress.

While your physical doors are heavily guarded, the Warden has spent years building psychological back doors out of your daily habits, routines, and environments. In the medical world, doctors call these "triggers," but we like to think of them as signs or superstitions. They're the Warden's ultimate predictive shortcuts gone completely off the rails.

The Guard/Warden is a world-class pattern-seeker, constantly trying to link point A to point B to predict a future attack. So, he creates these rules by taking a high-definition snapshot of a past flare-up and overprotectively connecting that pain to whatever happened to be nearby; a specific sight, a sound, or even a time of day. Once that link is ingrained in your nerves, your brain stops waiting for your body to send a physical report. It just follows its new, superstitious manual: if you see the sign, trigger the alarm. This is why you can feel your muscles ache before you even move.

Visual Superstitions

I (Hayley) am not superstitious. But my brain is a little stitious because when I see something heavy begging to be picked up, I instantly feel the start of a migraine at the back of my head, a painful preventative strike against almost certain future pain.

This has got to be one of the most counterintuitive glitches in human biology. Isn't it ironic that your brain creates a small amount of pain now to prevent what it thinks will be a massive amount of pain later?

It's like a security system that burns the house down the second it detects a suspicious shadow, just so a burglar can't get in. A case in which the cure is worse than the disease.

My migraine was likely never a sign that I'd done something wrong; it was a sign that my brain was using its backseat driver privilege and slamming on the imaginary brake pedal for a tiny speed bump a mile down the road.

The Nocebo Effect

To see how just a thought can hijack your physical biology, let's look at one of the most extreme medical cases ever recorded. Mr. A's experience is the ultimate example of something scientists call the Nocebo Effect. If the Placebo Effect is the notion that just believing something is good for you can make you feel better, the Nocebo Effect is its deeply pessimistic counterpart. The Nocebo Effect is the notion that just believing something is bad for you can make you feel worse.

In 2007, a 26-year-old man known in medical literature as Mr. A was a participant in a clinical trial for a new antidepressant. He was drowning in a severe depressive episode, desperate for relief, but the trial medication didn't seem to be working. So when he was hit by a sudden wave of overwhelming despair, he decided to end his life.

He walked into his kitchen, grabbed his clinical trial medication, and swallowed all twenty-nine capsules left in the bottle, setting the empty plastic container down on the counter. To his brain, that empty bottle was now a signed death warrant, a visual guarantee that twenty-nine lethal doses of a powerful chemical were currently dissolving in his stomach.

He regretted his decision almost immediately. Terrified, he rushed to the hospital, but by the time he reached the emergency room, his body was already acting on the visual command he had given it. His blood pressure plummeted to a life-threatening 80/40, and he was breathing rapidly in a state of full physical shock. He was pale, lethargic, and his heart was racing. Even after doctors pumped four liters of intravenous fluids into him, his body refused to stabilize.

The medical team was baffled until the clinical trial's lead researcher rushed into the ER, checked the records, and dropped a bombshell: Mr. A was in the control group. Those twenty-nine capsules weren't a lethal dose of medicine. They were just sugar. The moment the doctor explained that the "poison" was actually a placebo, a miracle happened. Within fifteen minutes, Mr. A's blood pressure and heart rate normalized, and he walked out of the hospital fully recovered.

To the "superstitious" mind of Mr. A, that empty pill bottle on his counter was a clear sign of danger. Though no toxic chemicals ever hit his bloodstream, his brain accepted that visual sign as a finished reality and started shutting down his body to prepare for the end.

Auditory Superstitions

Auditory superstitions live in the space where your brain attaches a dark piece of Lore to a specific sound. Hearing the ping of a work email after hours or the voice of a person associated with causing you high stress can trigger an instant cascade of overprotection in which your brain doesn't just loop the thought (Rumination); it also makes the consequences feel life-altering (Catastrophizing), turns a slight tension in your back into a full-blown cramp (Magnification), and makes you feel like there's nothing you can do to stop the cycle (Helplessness).

It's Pavlovian. Your brain is a master pattern-recognizer. So, if a specific sound (the ping) were ever followed by a high-cortisol event (a reprimand, a crisis, a conflict), even just a few times, your brain tags that audio frequency as dangerous, creating a neural shortcut. Before your conscious mind can even process the sound, the Warden has already executed the defensive playbook.

Temporal Signs and Superstitions

But the Warden doesn't just keep his eyes and ears open for physical sights and sounds; he also keeps a meticulous eye on the clock.

If you find yourself hitting an immovable wall of exhaustion every day at, say, 3:00 PM sharp, regardless of how much sleep you got, you are responding to a temporal superstition. Because of Hebb's Law, (the rule that neurons that fire together, wire together), the neurons representing 3:00 PM and the neurons representing total system shutdown have become a single, high-speed circuit.

While every human has a tiny biological dip in energy in the afternoon, your brain has catastrophized yours. It's not reacting to what you are doing; it's reacting to *when it is*, because the lore says that 3:00 PM is when your brain declares, "give me couch or give me death!"

Temporal superstitions are the time rules you unconsciously live by. For example, insisting that you can't drink a small sip of tea after 4:00 PM because it will keep you up all night is a temporal superstition. Just like the 3:00 PM wall, it's just neurons that have learned to fire together. Essentially, you have wired the clock to the alarm, and now your brain reacts to time, not caffeine.

That's why the moment you take a sip at 4:05 PM, or heaven forbid, 6:00 PM, your brain has already decided you're staying awake until dawn. When the reality is that even if you drink that cup at 6:00 PM, a cup of tea is like a small flashlight. By 10:00 PM, having a portion of that caffeine left is like having a flashlight with a dying battery. It's physically on, but it doesn't have the power to light up the stadium or keep you from seeing the darkness of sleep.

The Feedback Loop

In the movie Groundhog Day, the main character, Phil Connors, is a disgruntled weatherman sent to cover a story he hates when he finds himself trapped in a glitch in reality where he is forced to relive the same day over and over. No matter how much he tries to escape, the clock resets, and he is back at the same 6:00 AM.

Phil is trapped in his own forecast, caught in the feedback loop of his cynicism. In this loop, his cynical attitude (the input) creates a miserable day (the output), which only makes him more cynical (the new input). It's like the cycle feeds itself.

Phil wakes up expecting the world to be cold and miserable. Because he acts on that cynicism, he treats people poorly, which ensures he has a miserable day. That misery then becomes the proof he needs to stay cynical the next morning. He is trapped because his own weather report provides the very evidence he needs to keep the storm going.

Your overprotective brain does the same thing with your body. It creates a biological Groundhog Day by turning its own protective actions into the very weather it's reporting on.

Instead of predicting snow or rain, your brain acts like a nervous weatherman constantly forecasting a physical threat with a forecast of pain. When this prediction is made, your muscles instantly tense in preparation for an expected blow. Inevitably, this constant bracing locks your tissues into a persistent state of high alert, choking off local blood vessels. With the pipeline restricted, a total blockade forms, leaving your Maintenance Crew (the parasympathetic system) stranded outside the area when they should be repairing and relaxing the site.

Because the Maintenance Crew is blocked, they can't haul away the trash of the natural chemical exhaust that builds up whenever a muscle is working.

That exhaust then sits in your tissues and turns the environment acidic. This eventually starts to burn and irritate your nerves, which sends a 10 out of 10 scream of pain back to your brain.

This is where the weatherman's logic kicks in. The Warden hears that scream and says, "See? My forecast was right! The storm is here!" He doesn't realize the "storm" he is reporting on is actually the result of the tense muscles he ordered five minutes ago. Like Phil Connors, your overprotective brain scares itself with its own report. And it uses that pain (the output) as the reason to brace even harder (the new input), ensuring the cycle never ends.

It's like a physical phoenix: you can fight the fear and burn it down a thousand times, but the pain will always rise right back up from its own ashes.

This might sound like a poetic observation, but in overprotective pain it becomes a biological reality. Every time you give in to an episode of pain, hiding away and freezing in anticipation of misery, your brain uses that retreat as proof that a disaster occurred. It then uses the remnants of that retreat to justify the next round of searchlights and sirens.

But here is the secret the Warden doesn't want you to know: A phoenix only rises if there are ashes to build from. The cycle is immortal only as long as you mistake the smoke of a protective simulation for the fire of a physical emergency.

But the phoenix of your pain starts to lose its power the moment you recognize it for what it is, a recycled forecast, not a current fact. By identifying your own subconscious superstitions and refusing to provide the fuel of further fear, you stop feeding the fire. You don't just burn the fear; you eventually clear the ashes, leaving nothing for the cycle to rise from.

The Survival Tax

But the cost of this recycled forecast isn't just felt in your nerves; it is billed directly to your energy reserves. In Chapter 5, we looked at the massive hidden tax of constant vigilance, and the deep emotional and physical fatigue that comes from keeping your inner Guard on a permanent wartime footing. But this perpetual defense doesn't just exhaust your mind; it charges a bill directly to your cells, driving your body into a state of metabolic bankruptcy.

Deep inside every cell in your body are tiny power plants called mitochondria. Their job is to produce adenosine triphosphate (ATP)—the currency your body uses for fuel. Normally, that currency is distributed fairly: some goes to movement, some to digestion, and a huge portion goes to your Maintenance Crew for cellular repair and recovery.

But when the Warden locks your brain into a survival loop, he completely hijacks the local power grid. Because your muscles are trapped in that constant state of guarding, they are burning through ATP at an unsustainable rate. Even though you might be lying perfectly still on the couch trying to rest, your cells are doing the metabolic work of a marathon runner just to keep you "safe" from a perceived threat.

To make matters worse, the nervous system itself is a massive energy hog. Keeping the internal alarms blaring requires a non-stop stream of power.

This is where your Maintenance Crew hits a double disaster. First, the constant physical guarding acts like a literal chokehold on your tissues, mechanically blocking the crew from getting into the area, and then the survival-mode loop creates a total energy deficit. Even if you could magically lift the physical blockade right now, the crew would still be left sitting in the dark. They have no tools, no resources, and no power to fix the walls or wash away the acidic chemical trash.

Your cells are quite literally running out of gas trying to protect you from a maybe, leaving your entire system metabolically overdrawn.

The Price of Our Lore

This metabolic exhaustion is not a random system failure; it is the direct biological consequence of a mind caught in a constant loop of catastrophic forecasting. This catastrophization cycle is your overprotective brain's survival-at-all-costs logic in action, but its most devastating work isn't just the pain it produces; it's the reality it replaces. When your brain accepts the lore of your own brokenness, it stops being a neutral protector and becomes a frantic forecaster as it starts treating every sign and superstition as an absolute truth.

This is the central paradox of the overprotective brain: in its desperate attempt to ensure survival, it bankrupts the very life it is trying to protect.

We often think of catastrophization as just worrying, but in the Prison, it acts as a mandatory survival tax. The Warden doesn't just think about the storm; he hikes up the energy usage and funnels your entire metabolic budget into the searchlights and the sirens. He locks your muscles in a protective chokehold until the environment turns acidic, effectively burning the furniture to keep the house warm. He is so busy bracing for a "maybe" that he has forgotten how to live in the "is."

This feedback loop ensures that your own biological Groundhog Day never ends. The more you brace, the more your tissues scream, and the more they scream, the more the weatherman points to the pain as proof that his catastrophic forecast was right. He is trapped in his own echo chamber; terrorized by a storm that he accidentally manufactured. By treating his own protective defenses as evidence of an outside threat, he ensures the alarm never turns off.

But if the pain is a preemptive strike and the fatigue is an unpaid tax, then the walls of your Prison are thinner than they appear. They were not built from permanent damage or irreversible biology. They were built from prediction. And what your brain learned to predict, it can learn to predict differently.

The original injury may be real. The tissue issue may even remain. But the cycle survives because of what the Warden predicts next. Whether the threat is real, exaggerated, or entirely imagined, the forecast becomes part of the prison.

The nail isn't in your foot; it's in the Warden's forecast.

Part IV
Inside the Prison

9

The Load-Bearing Brain

When Responsibility Becomes Pain

"We don't see things as they are, we see them as we are."
—Anaïs Nin

If you could drop someone from 1901 into the middle of your typical Monday, they probably wouldn't be as shocked by your car or the smartphone as they would be overwhelmed by your pace. Their world was built around the rising and setting of the sun, physical chores, and natural pauses. In our world, those natural boundaries have largely disappeared. Today, we process more information in twenty-four hours than someone at the turn of the century did in a year.

We are basically living through a global experiment in hyper-vigilance. Our biology is ancient hardware trying to keep up with a high-speed data stream that never actually stops. Researchers have found that the normal level of internal noise and anxiety carried by a typical young person today actually exceeds the levels that would have landed someone in a clinical ward in the 1950s. Having traded intervals of work for a life that is always on, our brains are constantly vibrating.

The parts of your brain that make you you, the parts that remember your first car, learned how to use an iPhone, and manage your retirement account are not the parts running the Warden's office. As we've seen, the Warden's office lies in the limbic system and the amygdala. These are the lower chambers of the fortress, what we might think of as the basement of the Inner Keep, biologically almost identical to the brains of humans who lived 50,000 years ago.

This means your brain is essentially split into two very different wings. Up in the Administrative Wing, your logical brain is incredibly fast at processing new facts and navigating the modern world. It's built for rapid adaptation and instant knowing; it understands exactly what a mortgage is, it knows that an unread email isn't a predator, and it can accept a new reality in a heartbeat.

Operating on an entirely different script is the high-security wing in the basement. Logic means nothing down here. Far removed from your conscious thoughts, this ancient system cares only about what it physically senses. You can read a new fact or force a positive thought all you want; the basement won't update its records. Instead, it demands a different currency: physical patterns and relentless repetition.

Think about what happens when you stay in a hotel. Your administrative wing looks around the bathroom and notes that the towels are to the right of the sink and the toilet paper is on the left, which means you logically know exactly where everything is.

But the next morning, when you're half-asleep, your hand automatically reaches to the right, exactly where the toilet paper is located in your house. Your logical brain has the map, but the Warden is still running the old script. This happens because your brain requires repeated successful *experiences* before it updates a physical movement. It doesn't care that you know you're in a hotel; it only cares about the thousands of times you reached to the right at home.

Here lies the temporal gap that defines overprotective pain. Your administrative wing operates in seconds, but your high security wing operates in seasons. Reading a book like this one, your logical brain can understand the false alarm in a heartbeat. But the Warden is still pacing the Watch Room, marking threats on a map that your logical brain knows is out of date. And offering him a better argument won't help. What he's waiting for is a new, consistent track record of safe, relaxed experience.

The Warden Doesn't Speak English (or any other heart language)

The Warden speaks the language of survival signals. His job is to watch your heart rate, your cortisol levels, and your muscle tension. He doesn't see the email from your boss that makes your stomach sink; instead, he only sees the spike in adrenaline and the way your shoulders creep up to your ears. For thousands of years, those physical signals only meant one thing: a predator was in the bushes.

Because his reactions are instinctual and baked into your DNA, he doesn't learn that a mortgage isn't lethal. In his world, anything that causes that much sustained stress must be a life-or-death situation. So he doesn't wait for the Council to explain that it's just a busy Monday. He immediately pulls the emergency override, armoring your body with pain or preparing you to run with anxiety.

This disconnect explains why you can sit comfortably in your favorite chair, logically knowing you are safe, while your back screams and your heart races. Your logical brain is living in the 21st century, but your protection system is still living in the Stone Age, reacting to every vibration of the stress you're carrying. He has no need to understand the modern world to lock the doors; he only needs to sense the smoke of your stress.

The Shift from Nerves to Soul

Up until now, we've been looking at the mechanics of the Fortress, the wiring of the Gatehouse, the geography of your brain maps, and the way the alarm system is designed to keep you safe. And with all that, it's easy to look at the biology of overprotective pain and see it as a technical problem to be solved. But your brain isn't a machine, and your protection system isn't against you. It's actually incredibly loyal, so loyal, in fact, that it doesn't just react to physical injury; it reacts to the entire experience of being you.

As we move deeper into the Prison, we are moving from the mechanics of the nerves to the experience of the soul. We are going to stop looking at the wiring and start looking at what the Warden is actually trying to save you from.

The Warden doesn't just smudge your maps for fun; he smudges them because he is trying to protect your very identity from the crushing pressures of the world in which you live. For most of us, the prison isn't built solely out of diseased tissue or inflamed organs. It's also built from the drive to be a perfect parent, the relentless demands of a career, or a deep-seated sense of duty that never lets us rest. Seeing the exhaustion and the pressure of these roles, the Warden decides that the only way to save you is to ground you with pain in order to shield you from the overwhelming weight of your own responsibilities.

Bearing this intense burden requires an immense amount of structural scaffolding. Think about what we are actually doing when we take it upon ourselves to manage every variable, predict every crisis, and guarantee everyone else's security. Without realizing it, we have assumed a level of control that belongs only to the Divine. We have climbed onto a throne of total accountability, operating under the unconscious delusion that the entire world will collapse if we stop holding it up.

Now, whether you believe in a literal Grand Architect or simply a brilliant natural order to the universe, the engineering reality remains the same: your frame was never designed to bear the weight of the world. You were built to participate in life, not to manufacture its final outcomes.

Trying to play the role of the ultimate protector forces your brain to interpret that psychological responsibility as a crushing, physical load. But relief starts the moment you trade the exhausting crown of the Executive for the humble posture of a Steward. Embracing stewardship allows your system to recognize that while you have a vital role to play, you are not the source of the results. This single cognitive shift signals to the amygdala that it is finally safe to stand down, acknowledging a beautiful, liberating truth: the world will keep turning even after you set the weight down.

The Weight You Bear

The Warden handles the heavy burden of your perceived control by treating it as a literal, physical weight you bear. To your ancient brain, there is no difference between the weight of the sky you're trying to keep from falling and the weight of a heavy stone you're forced to carry. In both cases, your brain predicts a structural failure. When you live with this God-sized complex of total responsibility, your brain triggers a process called **protective guarding.**

This is an instinctual armor. You've felt it before: your brow furrows as you scan for problems, your jaw clenches, and you hold your breath. This is your brain turning your soft tissues into a shield to protect your vitals. In the world of our ancestors, this was a short-term win; it protected them during a fall or a fight. But in a world where the impact is a continuous stream of modern demands, it never stops.

Because the pressure you feel is constant, your nervous system starts treating your life like a structural load that your body has to permanently carry. It doesn't just pick a joint at random to lock down. Instead, it identifies the part of your biology that is already under the most strain, whether that is physical, emotional, or symbolic, and it pulls the emergency brake right on it.

Far from trying to punish or hurt you, this functional intervention is a desperate safety measure; a choice by the Warden to ground your most overtaxed system before the entire frame gives out.

For example, if you are a singer whose entire identity is tied to your voice, and you are terrified of giving a bad performance, the Warden probably won't make your big toe hurt. Instead, he might pull the brake on your vocal folds or your diaphragm, not to ruin your career, but to "save" you from the high-stakes terror of singing poorly. And if you are a writer under a crushing deadline, the Warden might not seize your lower back. Instead, he might trigger the fire alarm in your wrists and hands, not to punish you for working, but to protect you from the relentless pressure of the deadline by making it physically impossible to type another word.

This is how your Prison comes to feel so deeply personal. Your system strategically identifies your specific load; whether it is the pressure of financial survival, an over-responsible role, or a cherished dream where the emotional stakes are high, and the fear of failure is too. Then it pulls the plug on the exact physical equipment you need to carry that weight. That's because in primitive logic, your desperate fear of failure is a warning of an incoming, devastating emotional blow. And because your brain cannot tell the difference between a shattered dream and a shattered bone, the ultimate act of protection is to physically disable you before the world can emotionally crush you.

The Symbolic Load

Your brain is incredibly literal. If you feel like you can't *stomach* a situation at work, your nervous system might actually slow down your digestion. If you feel like you are *carrying* the weight of the world on your shoulders, your trapezius muscles will eventually feel like they are made of concrete.

This is your amygdala using your body to express the truth of your environment, turning your metaphorical load into a physical reality to force you to pay attention.

And this isn't just a theory; in her landmark study, "*Does Rejection Hurt?*", Dr. Naomi Eisenberger, a leading neuroscientist at UCLA, changed the way we understand the brain when she proved that it doesn't just feel social rejection, it processes it using the same neural hardware as a physical blow to the body.

In her study, she discovered that the Anterior Cingulate Cortex (ACC), the part of your brain that tells you how much a physical injury hurts, is the exact same area that lights up when you experience social rejection or emotional distress.

So, when you feel pushed aside at work, blindsided by a partner, or crushed by the weight of responsibility, your ACC registers that as a physical threat. Since it doesn't have a separate emotional folder to store these feelings, it sounds the same alarm it would use if you had broken a bone. Your nervous system responds with its only survival protocol: it armors your frame and locks your joints to prevent further injury. In the eyes of your biology, a broken heart and a broken leg are processed in the same office.

The Responsibility Hip

In my (Hayley's) case, the amygdala targeted my right hip. For a season, I struggled with crippling hip pain that didn't make any sense. Imaging didn't explain it. Rest didn't resolve it. The pain seemed out of proportion to anything happening in the joint itself.

Then I looked at the literal mechanics of the joint itself: the hip is the epicenter of forward motion, the very pivot point that allows us to step out and maintain balance. By locking it down, my nervous system was strategically disabling the equipment I was using to run myself into the ground. Since my system classified my frantic pace as a threat to my survival, it simply took away my ability to keep marching.

What I was experiencing wasn't just a localized hip strain; it was a textbook biological crisis of alignment that anyone carrying a heavy load will recognize. Since our brains require deep harmony between what we believe and how we actually live, when we step out of our depth and try to carry the weight of the world, our biology treats that internal conflict as a literal hazard.

But the shift toward my healing started when I stopped trying to be the source of everyone's stability and started seeing myself as a participant in a much larger order.

To see yourself in this light, it helps to assume a posture of surrender. I have found that whether through meditation or a quiet, outward-focused dialogue like prayer, the act of vocalizing my burdens to a space beyond myself has a measurable effect on my nervous system. It moves my brain out of a problem-solving loop and into a state of receptive trust. By acknowledging a reality larger than my own immediate crisis, I give my body permission to stop bracing for a fight it was never meant to win alone.

This shift didn't just change my mind; it began to signal to my nervous system that it was finally safe to let go. I didn't know it yet, but I was beginning to lay the groundwork for a total system reset.

The Speed of Safety

This internal surrender is a massive turning point, but your biology does not automatically keep pace with your breakthroughs. You might experience a profound moment of peace during prayer or meditation on a Friday night, yet wake up on Saturday morning with the exact same physical ache.

This frustrating delay happens because your breakthrough occurred entirely within the Administrative Wing. Your logical mind can accept a new reality in a heartbeat, but as we saw with the hotel bathroom, the Basement Wing operates on an entirely different timeline. It doesn't speak English, it doesn't care about your new spiritual insights, and it refuses to rewrite its security protocols overnight. While your conscious mind can choose surrender in a second, the Warden requires a season of consistent evidence before he will safely stand down.

Operating on this historical lag, the basement continues to broadcast an electrical stay-away order long after the initial threat has passed. The Warden keeps his hand firmly on the panic button because, to his primitive survival logic, a single moment of quiet reflection hasn't proven that the environment is genuinely safe. This is why merely understanding the emotional root of your pain does not immediately change the physical reality of feeling it.

To alter the signal, you can't just argue with the basement; you have to offer it physical proof. When you choose to move, step forward, or enter the exact environments the Warden is guarding, and nothing falls apart, your nervous system finally receives the data it needs. But an overzealous bodyguard will never stand down because you show him a new line of logic; he only steps aside when he experiences safety over time.

This negotiation is inherently slow because the Warden is an obsessive record-keeper. He ignores how peaceful you feel right now to focus instead on the persistent stress patterns you established over the last six months. This lag is exactly why the timing of your symptoms can feel so utterly irrational, and why your body can still scream at you on a lazy Saturday morning while you are trying to enjoy your pancakes. Your brain is just executing its programming, fiercely bracing for a threat it assumes is still lurking just around the corner.

The Science of the Groove

This ability to anticipate a threat before it even arrives is rooted in the Guard/Warden's greatest superpower: he is a master at spotting patterns. If you spend three months tightening your shoulders because of a crushing deadline at work, the Warden doesn't just see a temporary stressor; he records a permanent security policy.

With every stressful repetition, he carves a physical groove into your brain's gray matter, linking your daily environment directly to your protection system. Eventually, the basement stops waiting for the actual anxiety to arrive; it just pre-loads the pain the moment it smells the familiar smoke of your morning routine. This is the exact mechanism by which a temporary, life-saving protection strategy hardwires itself into a permanent learned pain response.

The Golfer in the Scanner

To see this groove in action, researchers studied two groups of golfers: one with over-protective back pain and another who were pain-free. They placed the participants in an fMRI scanner, and gave them a singular instruction:

"Don't move. Just imagine yourself swinging your club."

When the healthy golfers imagined their swing, their brains performed a high-speed mental rehearsal. Even though they were lying perfectly still, the *movement* centers responsible for their back, shoulders, and hips fired in a precise sequence. To the nervous system, there was no difference between the thought and the act; the brain was literally running the software for the movement, firing the exact neural circuits required for the swing.

This is the groove in action. Your brain isn't just preparing for an event in the future; it is performing a high-fidelity simulation in the present.

For the golfers in pain, this means the Warden didn't even need them to pick up a club to start the protection protocol. He just needed them to think about the swing, and he immediately triggered the pain signal to stop the action he's already seeing play out in your motor cortex.

To the researchers, the data showed a brain that had completely reclassified the golf swing. It was no longer an athletic feat to be practiced; it was a threat to be managed.

This study shattered the traditional medical model of pain because it proved that the brain doesn't need a physical stimulus to trigger a full-scale emergency response. It doesn't even need you to try to move. It only needs you to think about moving.

The Emotional Weight

If Chapter 8 showed how the brain becomes a historian, obsessed with what has already happened, we now see the brain as an architect actively trying to build a body capable of withstanding the weight of the world. This bridge between a conscious thought and a physical reaction is orchestrated by the limbic system (the Inner Keep), your brain's emotional headquarters.

Think of your limbic system as a master translator sitting between the conscious mind and the physical body. Its job is to scan the environment for high-stakes signals and convert them into biological action. It doesn't store responsibilities like cold, clinical files; it stores them like weighted experiences. So, when your brain processes the pressure of your unending inbox, the silent friction in your marriage, or the fear of being found out as a fraud, your limbic system doesn't see a workable to-do list; it sees a survival threat.

When you say something like, "I'm completely overwhelmed," or say you're feeling "crushed" by a deadline, your incredibly literal brain doesn't realize these are figures of speech used to describe a stressful week. Instead, it interprets the emotional gravity of the situation as a physical demand for resources.

The moment your limbic system decides that the cost of failure is rising, it issues a physical command: reinforce the pillars. It doesn't wait for your hands to pick up a literal heavy box; it triggers the motor cortex to armor your spine and hips in anticipation of the weight it thinks is being carried. This is the point where a heavy heart becomes back pain: the moment an abstract thought is translated into a concrete, physical command to survive.

The Vacation Flare

This architectural prep work explains a frustratingly common phenomenon, what doctors call **the let-down effect,** often experienced as a vacation flare. It's the pattern where someone pushes through intense stress, only to get sick or collapse the moment they finally stop.

While the load of your life is active, your system stays in high alert, your brain flooding your body with stress hormones like cortisol and adrenaline, which act as a powerful chemical mask for pain. In this high-alert state, as we've said, your brain deprioritizes maintenance signals in favor of survival signals. That means that it doesn't matter if your back hurts; the show must go on.

But the minute the deadline passes and the pressure drops, the chemical masking fades. The system stands down, adrenaline recedes, and your brain is suddenly forced to process what it has been ignoring for weeks. Your body has been carrying tension and strain, but your brain has been keeping it in the background so you can function. When the pressure lifts, that background signal gets brought forward.

And while the external stressor may be gone, the pattern of protection can stay if your system has learned bracing. In that case, what started as a response to pressure becomes a habit of building up your defenses, in which your brain starts to treat similar movements as a potential threat, even when the original strain is over.

This is the hangover of overprotective pain. Your responsibility hip doesn't care that the deadline has passed; it's still vibrating with the ghost of the pressure you just survived. Because the Warden is an obsessive record-keeper who is still counting the costs of a battle that ended yesterday, your pain persists.

The Biological Budget

This persistent guarding doesn't just hurt, it is bankrupting you.

Neuroscientist Dr. Lisa Feldman Barrett describes this as **allostasis**, the brain's way of managing your body budget. While you may see perfectionism or responsibility as personality traits, the Warden sees them as high-priced line items on your balance sheet. Every moment you spend guarding against the invisible gravity of your life, he's writing a check your biology can barely cash.

To prevent what he perceives as a systemic collapse, the Warden acts as a predictive governor, putting the entire system on a permanent, high-security lockdown. And this is where the math catches up with you: In his desperate attempt to save the business, the Warden is actually the one bankrupting you.

By diverting every ounce of your energy into security, guarding, hyper-vigilance, and constant pain signals, he leaves nothing in the budget for maintenance. He is like a CEO who spends the company's last dollar on a private army while the factory roof is caving in. He thinks he's saving the business, but his overspending on protection is the very thing keeping your system in the red.

The Micromanaging CEO

A brain running in a deficit behaves a lot like that panicked CEO when the budget is in the red.

When a company is thriving, profits are high, and customers are happy, the CEO doesn't sweat the small stuff. He doesn't notice if an employee takes a long lunch or if a report is ten minutes late. The company has a surplus, so minor infractions are ignored.

But when a business starts to fail, when customers are unhappy, or the budget is in the red, the boss's personality shifts. He stops just looking at the big picture and starts micromanaging every employee. He demands audits of every department: the knees, the digestion, the lower back, and during an audit, you will always find something wrong.

When the CEO senses a problem, he's more apt to notice Bill taking a slightly longer lunch break or Nancy coming in late every other day. In a healthy year, these were non-issues. But in a crisis, the CEO loses his sense of proportion.

This is exactly how an overprotective brain manages a body under threat. In this condition, pain isn't a sign of a new injury; it's the result of a panicked CEO who has lost the ability to distinguish a late report from a total corporate collapse.

The Anatomy of the Invisible

When the CEO triggers these internal audits, he doesn't just look at random data. He targets the exact physical structures where you are carrying your heaviest psychological weight.

To dismantle this lockdown, you have to identify which of these three specific cargo loads your body is currently trying to brace against:

1. The Load of Responsibility

Responsibility is the most common modern load because it's the standard price of admission for adulthood. We aren't just responsible for ourselves; we become the structural support for everyone else. And there is a particular weight that goes along with being the load-bearing member of a system.

To the Warden, being the person everyone relies on is a physical mandate for absolute rigidity. So, he identifies the structural support beams of your body, the hips, the lower back, and the pelvis, and reinforces them. In his literal logic, a flexible beam is a collapsing beam. If the people around you are heavy, your foundation must be frozen to keep them upright.

Over time, the brain automates this guarding. Your responsibility hip becomes a permanent fixture, long after the children have moved out or the business has been sold, because your brain has forgotten how to be anything other than a support beam.

2. The Load of Perfectionism

Perfectionism is often misunderstood as a personality trait, but to the limbic system, it's taken as a high-stakes evaluation of threat. If you believe that a single mistake will lead to rejection, failure, or a loss of status, your brain operates in a state of constant trial, creating a state of micro vigilance. It tightens the smaller, stabilizing muscles, the ones that control fine motor skills and posture, so that you are always ready to perform. Thus creating a brittle, fragile kind of strength.

When a mistake feels like a catastrophe, your brain simply outlaws rest. Instead, the system redlines twenty-four hours a day, sending a restless, traveling pain that mimics the constant, exhausting hum of an overtaxed engine.

3. The Load of Grief and Shame

Grief and shame could be the heaviest loads because they are often carried in secret. While responsibility pulls us tight to support others, grief and shame often cause the system to protect our core.

Your nervous system's response to internal pain is often an inward tightening of your musculature. This is where we see the grief-stricken back or the shoulders of shame as your brain attempts to physically curl around the heart and the gut to protect the most vulnerable parts of the body. This creates a permanent state of flexion, a literal physical closing of your body. Even after the initial shock of a loss or the sting of a secret has faded, your body stays in its protective huddle, waiting for a second blow that might never even come.

Moving Beyond the Load

Recognizing which load your body is responding to is the first step in rewriting the security file. The reason traditional physical therapy often fails for overprotective cases is that you can't force a responsibility hip to relax through mechanical stretching alone, nor can you strengthen your way out of a perfectionist back.

These aren't always mechanical failures. Often, they are functional choices made by a Warden who is still bracing for impact. By this point, the only way to change your system's verdict is through evidence.

This doesn't mean movement is useless; in fact, movement is the only way out. But the goal of the exercises in the following chapters isn't just to lengthen your hamstrings; it is to provide neurological evidence to your body that the Warden can return to being Captain of the Guard again. When you move a locked joint in a safe, controlled way, you're showing him that the cornerstone can shift without the house falling down. That means, you aren't just stretching a muscle; you are renegotiating a security policy.

The Architecture of Protection

Healing isn't about forced change but returning to our original design. We were built for cycles of high-intensity action followed by deep, restorative rest. But when the demands of our lives exceed our capacity to rest, our biology interprets that strain as a mandate to lock down and protect our core.

Your pain is not a sign that your body is failing you; it's the ultimate expression of your system's fierce loyalty to you, the result of a system that has decided that guarding your frame is the only way to keep your head above water.

By identifying these loads, you can learn to stop being a victim of unexplained pain and start becoming a witness to your own protection. No longer fighting a malfunction, you can observe the sophisticated management decision made by a brain just trying to balance a budget under immense pressure.

While we aren't here to tear down the walls of a fortress designed to keep you safe, recognizing the architecture of your makeshift prison allows you to stop leaning against the alarm. Understanding why you are braced gives your nervous system permission to stand down.

So now, we've seen how the foundation was laid and how the pillars were braced, now, we have to look at the rest of the internal environment, the atmosphere of anxiety and the heavy fog of depression, that completes the experience of life inside the cell.

10

The Projection Room

How Anxiety Traps Your Brain in a Fictional Script

"The soul becomes dyed with the color of its thoughts."

-Marcus Aurelius

In the 1998 film The Truman Show, the protagonist lives in a world that is, unbeknownst to him, a massive, meticulously constructed movie set. Every person he meets is an actor; every storm is a special effect; every horizon is a painted wall. For thirty years, Truman Burbank's brain does exactly what yours and mine are designed to do: accept the world as it is presented. He doesn't question the sky because it looks like a sky to him. He doesn't question his paralyzing fear of the ocean because he was trained by a scripted childhood tragedy to believe the water is a death trap.

Truman's entire reality is a beautifully orchestrated illusion, manufactured by a director sitting in a high-tech control room, pulling levers to manipulate his emotions and keep him from ever leaving the set.

Your brain's threat-detection system is already a master prediction machine; as we've seen, it creates the sensation of pain to protect you from what it predicts is happening to your body right now. But anxiety takes this predictive machinery and forces the Warden to step into the projection booth. Acting as a rogue director, he shoots a massive, terrifying disaster movie about your entire future, and then forces you to watch it on repeat.

Welcome to the Projection Room.

This shift from predicting immediate physical danger to projecting a future catastrophe fundamentally changes your internal tracking system.

At the center of the problem sits your Sergeant of the Gate (Thalamus), the executive in charge of your body's internal sorting office. It is his job to act as the ultimate Sorting Clerk—the one responsible for sorting through millions of incoming sensory inputs, filing away the background noise, and only handing you the urgent, high-priority signals. In a predictable, regulated brain, the Sergeant ruthlessly silences the static. He ignores the minor, normal twinge in your lower back, the ambient hum of the room, and the vague worry about next week.

But **anxiety fundamentally changes the Sergeant's marching orders.** Because anxiety convinces the brain that the future is entirely unsafe, it forces your nervous system to treat every single background ripple in your body as an imminent threat. It demands that your brain pay hyper-focused, panicked attention to the very static it's supposed to ignore.

This is exactly how pain and anxiety form their devastating partnership. With the director in the Projection Room screaming about imaginary disasters, the Sergeant of the Gate is forced to abandon his post. The internal filter breaks down, and the gates are left wide open.

Suddenly, your brain loses its ability to decide what doesn't matter.

Without the ability to prioritize information, your brain suffers a profound security breach. Every single incoming signal—an ambiguous email from your boss, a slight shift in your physical symptoms, a stray thought about your financial future—is treated with the exact same level of high-alert urgency. The floods rush in, and every minor background alert is treated like a maximum-priority executive order from the Warden.

When your brain can no longer accurately calculate what is safe and what is dangerous, it defaults to a brutal, evolutionary rule of thumb: assume everything is a catastrophe until proven otherwise.

To cope with this overwhelming flood of unfiltered data, your brain's internal director pulls a new lever. He stops tracking the physical reality of the room you're sitting in and starts running endless, high-budget, worst-case scenarios. What if this flare-up never ends? What if I lose my job? What if I try that new therapy and it ruins me?

Your nervous system, desperately trying to predict an unpredictable future, starts manufacturing its own terrifying scripts in order to keep you safe.

Muting the Live Feed

When the Warden takes over the projection booth, he doesn't just change the view; he alters what your brain is physically capable of perceiving, turning your inner theater into a high-stakes Alfred Hitchcock film, and trapping you in a psychological thriller where the tension is manufactured entirely by what *might* happen next. By locking your focus onto this oncoming disaster, the Warden blinds you to the actual reality of the room you are standing in.

Brain scanners caught this precise phenomenon in real-time. Researchers placed participants inside an fMRI machine and delivered a small, predictable, completely painless pulse of heat to their skin. Then, they gave the participants a single warning: "In a moment, we might give you a much bigger hit."

The second the participants started expecting the big hit, their brain activity radically shifted. The areas responsible for handling raw, objective sensation, the live feed from the body, were instantly muted, leaving the brain with no way to register that the present moment was actually safe. In that silence, the Director in the control room took over, over-interpreting every tiny internal ripple and turning a normal background hum into a full-blown siren.

This is the Projection Room in action. When you're trapped in a cycle of overprotective anxiety, your brain stops filtering the world for you, and the ordinary, uneventful moments feel completely overwhelming. A simple question from a spouse feels like an interrogation; the normal chaos of a grocery store feels like a war zone. Contrary to popular belief, you aren't being difficult, and your character hasn't changed; you're just irritable because your brain is failing to process the reality of the room you're standing in while it's locked onto a disaster film about the future.

And once your brain starts sounding the alarm for possibilities instead of real-time events, the siren has no address: it wails, but there's nowhere to send the medics. Like a guard drilling for a fight that never arrives, this anticipatory anxiety strikes at shadows just to prove it's ready. Obviously, if you treat that alarm the way you treat structural pain, resting it, bracing it, protecting it, you end up treating empty air. Whether or not a tissue issue is present, anxiety cannot be resolved by treating it like a local injury. The forecasting system itself must relearn how to listen to the live feed again.

The Fuel for the Forecast

To understand how this forecasting engine completely hijacks you, we have to separate the physical alarm from the psychological thriller. While pain may involve a specific physical coordinate, your stiff back or your aching knee, anxiety is the Warden defending a concept. It is protection without a physical location, and because it has no location, it has no limit.

A physical sensation, like a bee sting, is a finite event. But your imagination can run twenty-four hours a day, scripting catastrophes without ever needing a real-world reason.

Think about it this way: the suffering you experience isn't caused solely by the physical sensation itself; it's also shaped by the script playing over it. Imagine, for a minute, if you could take a Magic Pill that instantly deactivated your brain's ability to project threat or anxiety. If you then broke your arm, you would still receive a physical signal; you would know your arm was damaged. But the suffering, the agonizing "oh no," the racing heart, the mental image of a ruined career, would not be there. The signal would lose its teeth. You would be aware of the sensation, but you would no longer be haunted by it.

It's natural to think of this relentless mental chatter as if it's just the background noise of our pain. But it's not. The hijacking of your attention isn't just a side effect of suffering; *it is the suffering.* We tend to think of anxiety as an abstract emotion, but in the Warden's world, it is a total takeover of the control room.

In my (Sam's) practice, this imaginary pill became a stark reality when I was treating a child with cerebral palsy and significant brain damage. One day, I drove up to his house, and he ran out to meet me, tripped, and bashed his face directly into the cement. He immediately jumped up and kept running and laughing. No tears, no fear. Because of the way his brain was wired, the physical signal of the impact never triggered the alarm of the Warden.

Now, that might look like a superpower, but it is actually a tragedy. This is the dark irony of our biology: If you felt no pain, no grief, and no anxiety, you would be in a world of hurt. We often treat these negative states like invaders to be eliminated, but they are actually the most sophisticated safety features ever designed.

The goal of healing isn't to become like my client and feel nothing. The goal is to realize that the extreme suffering you feel is actually useful protective machinery being run at the wrong time (or run too many times.) Your Warden is just a dedicated employee who is currently terrified by his own imagination, trying to protect you from a face-plant that isn't happening.

But because that disaster is only playing out in your mind, your brain has to look at any physical sensations it can find for evidence. With no real-world enemy to fight, it grabs hold of a sudden stomach cramp, a dull ache, or a wave of nausea, and uses it to validate panic.

And the irony is this: the Warden isn't just finding these symptoms, he's actively manufacturing them. When the energy meant for healthy digestion is hijacked by the projection booth, your stomach knots up. Adding fuel to the fire, the Warden then looks at these physical distress signals and shouts, "See? I told you we were in trouble!" And like a mad conspiracy theorist pointing at a shadow he cast himself, he uses the physical byproducts of his own false alarms as the ultimate proof to keep the movie running.

In anxiety, your forecasting engine is completely outrunning your physical reality—your mind screaming at 8,000 RPMs, while you are just sitting on your couch. Because the Warden is reacting to a disaster in a simulated future, your nervous system is already living on Friday afternoon while your physical body is still standing in the peace of Sunday morning.

This is what neuroscientists call **Meta-protection**: the brain protecting its own ability to protect. In this, the Warden makes a radical strategic pivot. He decides that being right about a real, present threat is less important than never being surprised by a potential one. He stops asking, "*Is this dangerous?*" and starts asking a much more haunting question: "*Could this become dangerous*?"

This is where most of us get stuck: we feel the physical knots in our stomach or the tension in our neck and try to treat them like a standard injury. But you cannot apply a localized solution to an anchor-less alarm. You cannot rehab a what-if. When your internal alarm system is patrolling a digital horizon, it isn't looking for a cure; it is looking for certainty. That endless search for certainty comes with a steep neurological tax, levied every time the brain fails its most basic job: sorting the mail.

When Everything Becomes Important

The problem with a high-definition projection booth is all the data it creates. In a healthy system, your brain acts like a fast-paced company with an efficient sorting clerk. Every piece of incoming information, whether it's a physical sensation or a stray thought, is quickly categorized and routed into one of three mail bins:

Priority Mail (Useful): This is actionable, real, and present. The stove is on. I have a deadline in an hour. My knee is actually swelling. This data requires a response.

Non-Actionable Mail (Neutral): This is subjective or socially filtered info that doesn't require immediate action. My boss looked tired during my presentation. It might rain tomorrow. That person didn't text me back. It's interesting, but it isn't an emergency.

Junk Mail (Noise): This is random, speculative, or purely generated by the projection booth. What if I lose my job and end up homeless? What if this chest tightness is a rare disease? In a healthy brain, this mail is sent straight to the shredder so it never reaches the executive desk.

But in the Prison of Anxiety, the sorting clerk has become a radical extremist. He stops using the shredder altogether and routes every piece of junk mail directly to the Warden's desk.

The problem isn't that your brain is detecting too much; it's that it has stopped deciding what matters. When your system treats a random what-if with the same urgency as a house fire, you end up living with the exhaustion of responding to a fleeting thought as if it were a legally binding subpoena.

When everything is given equal weight, nothing can be processed correctly. The system never resolves anything because it never stops escalating. This is how the Warden sustains the narrative: a passing thought becomes an active threat, a vague sensation becomes physical evidence, and the body stops reacting to what is actually happening, reacting instead to what has been labeled important.

In 1983, a Soviet early-warning satellite falsely reported that five American nuclear missiles were heading for Moscow. The software—the automated sorting clerk of the military—had suffered a spectacular classification error: it had mistaken innocent sunlight glinting off the tops of clouds for the fiery exhaust of rocket engines. Because its algorithm was tuned to be hyper-reactive rather than accurate, it promoted a neutral atmospheric phenomenon into a maximum-priority, impeding global catastrophe.

The officer on duty, Stanislav Petrov, saved the world by refusing to react like a Warden and, instead, was the Captain of the Guard we all needed. He looked past the screaming screens, looked at the quiet room around him, and realized the system was panicking over background noise. This is exactly what an anxious brain does. It catches a harmless flash of light—a random thought or a strange physical sensation—and plays the apocalypse soundtrack over it. Healing is developing the capacity to look at the screen, look at the room, and recognize that your system is just looking at a reflection on the clouds.

The Cost of Misclassification

When the sorting clerk fails, and junk mail is promoted to priority, your system triggers the exact process we broke down in Chapter 8: rumination. But looking at it through the lens of the sorting office shows its true neurological cost. Because the Guard turned Warden has accepted a speculative what-if as an active threat, he demands a solution. But you cannot fight a ghost, and you cannot fix a fictional script with more thinking.

This is the ultimate loop of effort without exposure. Your brain is working with the intensity of an Olympic athlete while standing perfectly still, replacing the live feed of reality with a replay of the projection. The moment you stop trying to solve the crisis in your imagination and return to the evidence of the room, you deprive the loop of its fuel. You stop trying to think your way out and finally let the real world prove the junk mail wrong.

This isn't just a metaphor; it is exactly how your neurology operates. In the field of Computational Psychiatry, a shift is happening in how we view anxiety. It's no longer seen as just too much stress. Our sorting office concept is what neuroscientists call **Precision Weighting.**

For decades, classic textbook science taught us that the brain operates like a mirror. The theory was that your eyes and ears gather raw data from the outside world, beam it into your skull, and your brain passively records it to create your reality. But the physical world is a chaotic, overwhelming torrent of sensory information. If your brain had to consciously process every single piece of raw data from scratch every second—the hum of a refrigerator, the texture of your clothes, the shifting shadows on a wall—your neural circuitry would suffer an immediate meltdown.

To survive, your brain evolved a brilliant shortcut. It doesn't look at the world to see what's there. It guesses.

In computational psychiatry, this is known as the Bayesian Brain model. Instead of waiting for data to come in, your brain uses your past experiences, memories, and deep-seated beliefs to build a high-definition simulation of what it expects to happen next.

Your brain projects its pre-existing templates onto your environment and only uses your senses to spot-check for mistakes. When there is a mismatch (when you expect a flat floor but your foot hits a dip) your brain experiences a Prediction Error. It flashes a biological red flag that says: "The simulation doesn't match the room. Wake up and pay attention."

To resolve this mismatch, your sorting clerk has to calculate probability. It must make a split-second choice: Which data stream should I trust more? My internal simulation, or the incoming raw data from the physical room? If the power suddenly goes out in your house, your sorting clerk instantly shelves its internal map of the room and treats the incoming raw data from your physical senses as maximum-priority mail, tuning in to every tiny creak in the floorboards.

In a landmark review, **Dr. Sonia Bishop** showed that anxiety is a computational deficit where the brain loses its ability to properly weigh uncertainty, leading the overprotective brain to treat every speculative possibility as a high-priority threat.

When this sorting office is operating under overprotective anxiety, it defaults to a permanent emergency protocol. The clerk stops evaluating mail based on actual facts and starts routing letters based entirely on a rigid, worst-case scenario policy manual. The mailbox becomes constantly overflowing with unshredded junk mail, and your brain's internal algorithm gets completely corrupted, losing the ability to separate a trivial event from a true catastrophe. Because your brain doesn't just respond to what is happening, it responds to what it believes the experience is worth, what it signals, and what it predicts. When that internal scale shifts, even neutral moments begin to carry weight they were never meant to hold.

To revoke this emergency protocol and force the system to reset, you can't just tell the clerk to relax. You have to actively disrupt the rulebook by manufacturing what cognitive scientists call a "**Safety Prediction Error.**"

For years, classical psychology assumed that the only way to quiet an overprotective brain was through a process called "habituation." The theory was simple: if you put yourself in a terrifying situation, like a crowded store, you had to sit there and wait until your panic completely burned itself out like a dying fire. If you left the store while your heart was still racing, the old thinking went, your brain would learn nothing.

But groundbreaking clinical research, led by psychologist Dr. Michelle Craske at UCLA, has completely reframed how the brain actually rewrites its threat templates. The breakthrough model is called **Inhibitory Learning**, and its core discovery is incredibly liberating: long-term healing doesn't require your fear to completely disappear while you are facing it. You don't have to wait for your heart to stop pounding or for the anxious junk mail to vanish from the desk.

Instead, the true goal of exposure is simply to orchestrate a deliberate, undeniable mismatch between the junk mail's terrifying prediction and the actual, real-time data of the room. You aren't trying to force your body to feel calm; you are trying to test the accuracy of the rumor.

If a piece of speculative junk mail predicts that entering a crowded store or testing your physical baseline will result in a total body collapse, you must let that red-stamped priority file sit on the Warden's desk unanswered while you step into the room and gather the live feed. You don't run, you don't brace, and you don't argue with the projection. You just look around.

So if the junk mail says: If we stay here, we will faint. But as you stand in the aisle, feeling highly anxious but remaining upright, your physical senses stream a completely contradictory reality back to the sorting office: The air is flowing. The floor is solid. We are still standing. No disaster has occurred.

This massive gap between the horror story contained in the junk mail and the boring reality your body is experiencing creates a profound computational shockwave. This sudden mismatch that forces your brain to register that its automated sorting system just suffered a spectacular misclassification is the Safety Prediction Error in action.

Rather than erasing the old threat files (since the brain rarely deletes memories entirely) this experience slams a brand-new, dominant rule down on top of them. The result is a giant sticky note left across the mailbox that reads: This situation feels like an emergency, but the live data shows it turns out to be perfectly safe.

Every single time you allow this mismatch to happen without fleeing or running a mental rescue script, you validate the live feed. You are retraining the the Sergeant of the Gate to trust the room over the rumors, teaching him that uncertainty isn't an incoming missile—it's just unclassified mail.

Which is why anxiety doesn't just change your thoughts, it changes the way your brain measures the world. It uses the exact same mechanics a master filmmaker uses to manipulate an audience.

Ultimately, this is the psychological art of the Red Herring. In whodunit thrillers like Knives Out, directors deliberately use misdirection to make us misclassify the innocent as dangerous. The camera will linger aggressively on a completely ordinary detail—a broken window or a muddy footprint—while the musical score swells with ominous tension.

Because the atmosphere dictates danger, your brain automatically labels that neutral detail as a threat, only for the final twist to reveal it was entirely harmless.

Anxiety is a director who relies entirely on these cheap editing tricks. It takes a completely neutral internal sensation or a random, passing thought, zooms the camera in way too close, and plays a horror soundtrack over it. Knowing that, we can tell you that healing isn't about running out of the theater; it's about learning to look at the screen, recognizing the red herrings for what they are, and realizing that the terrifying atmosphere is just an illusion generated by a hyper-reactive booth.

The Beautiful Mind Strategy

There is a powerful illustration of this in the film, *A Beautiful Mind* which depicts the life of the Nobel Laureate John Nash. Nash suffered from schizophrenia, meaning his projection booth was running a literal spy thriller twenty-four hours a day. He saw people who weren't there and heard voices plotting against him.

For years, Nash tried to fix the hardware through heavy medication that numbed his entire life. When that failed, he tried to argue with the plot, using logic to prove the hallucinations weren't real. Neither worked. The projection just kept playing in high definition.

The turning point in the story, and the secret to his recovery, came at the end of the film. A colleague asks Nash if the hallucinations are gone. Nash glanced over his shoulder at three figures standing in the hallway, people only he could see, and said, "No, they're not gone. And maybe they never will be. But I've gotten used to ignoring them, and I think, as a result, they've given up on me."

In that moment, Nash performed the ultimate executive act: he moved his horror movie of a script straight to the junk mail bin. He realized he couldn't make it stop playing, but he could choose not to audition for a role in it. He stopped arguing with the spies and simply started ignoring them.

This is the exact intersection where the projection booth and the sorting office collide. When you are caught in the grip of anxiety, your internal sorting clerk panics and drops speculative scripts straight onto the Warden's desk. And the moment the Warden holds that fictional disaster in his hands, he feels he has no choice but to act it out, putting you center stage in a crisis that only exists on paper.

But as Nash proved, you don't need a perfectly quiet mind to have a quiet life. You just need to have a better sorting clerk. The junk mail of your imagination might never stop coming, but you can choose to recognize a speculative "what-if" and send it straight to the shredder before it ever triggers the Warden's alarms. Healing starts when you stop playing the lead actor in a manufactured drama and start acting as the gatekeeper who decides what actually makes it to the desk.

When you reclaim this executive power, choosing the live feed of reality over the projections of a terrified mind, your nervous system finally returns to its original, healthy design, and you step out of the hyper-reactive prison and back into a fortress designed for freedom.

And if you want to see what a lifetime of running that healthy baseline actually looks like in human flesh, you only have to look at my (Hayley's) eighty-five-year-old father.

The Cowboy Baseline

My father is a lifelong cowboy who still spends his days running a working ranch, throwing heavy hay bales, and climbing underneath massive, rusting tractors to wrench on their chassis. On the weekends, he barrel races all over the West Coast. And if you don't know what that is, it's a high-speed, high-impact, razor-sharp sport dominated almost entirely by women in their twenties. And he doesn't just participate; he regularly beats them.

Physically, an eighty-five-year-old body has unavoidable structural changes. Still, helpful Pain may still occasionally alert him to the limits of those tissues, but his nervous system has never learned to turn those signals into Overprotective Pain. If you put his spine or his knees into an MRI machine, you would undoubtedly find the standard wear-and-tear, the thinning cartilage, and the arthritic baselines that decades of hard ranch work and breaking horses naturally carve into the human body. By all textbook definitions of structural change, his system should be screaming.

But it isn't. He moves with a mostly unbothered fluid strength because his brain operates on the exact opposite baseline of an overprotective brain.

When my dad approaches a heavy tractor or mounts a horse, his sorting clerk doesn't intercept his physical intentions with a high-budget horror script. His brain doesn't scream: "What if your L4 disc herniates? What if you break a hip out here alone? What if this horse takes a bad step and ruins your remaining years?"

Because his internal volume knob, the gain control of his nervous system, is perfectly calibrated, his Sergeant of the Gate treats the ambient physical sensations of being eighty-five as harmless, non-actionable background noise. His brain looks at his long history of capability, spot-checks the live feed of the immediate present, and calculates an overwhelming probability of safety. It completely shreds the speculative junk mail of "what-if" before it ever hits the Guard's desk.

As a result, his system grants him full, uninhibited access to his physical power. The Sentinels of his fortress remain at ease because they aren't wasting precious neurological bandwidth patrolling for a crisis that hasn't happened yet. His soul, echoing the ghost of Marcus Aurelius, is dyed entirely in the color of real-time capability, not forecasted catastrophe.

Returning to the Council Chamber

Ultimately, you do not need to rewrite your history, fix your hardware, or guarantee an unpredictable future to find peace. You simply have to change which room is running your life. The horror scripts, the red herrings, the overflowing junk mail of an overprotective brain; they will likely keep arriving at the gates. But their power depends entirely on your compliance.

Like John Nash, you can choose to let the spies stand in the hallway without giving them a seat at the table. Like my father, you can rule from a baseline of safety, trusting the live feed of the immediate present over the speculative horror movies of a terrified Warden. The doors to your original fortress are open. Step off the movie set, quiet the theater, and return to the Council Chamber where your soul can finally be dyed in the color of real-time capability.

Part V

The Prison Returns to a Fortress

11

The Language of Safety

Rewriting the Script

"A man who cannot distinguish between imagination and reality is bound to suffer."
— Bertrand Russell

In the final act of The Truman Show, his life reaches a pivotal point. After thirty years of unknowingly living inside a massive televised set designed to imitate ordinary life, Truman starts to notice the seams. A light fixture labeled Sirius falls from a clear blue sky. Rain falls in one spot only, directly over his head. The same three people walk past his office in a repetitive, timed loop, and the simulation starts to crack.

For Truman, the discovery of these anomalies is the beginning of freedom. In a matter of minutes, he stops believing in the projection because the evidence no longer adds up. He realizes his "prison" is actually just a set with stagehands, wires, and lighting cues. And once he sees the anomalies, the fear that kept him paralyzed on that island for three decades loses its authority.

From Prisoner to Observer

To occupy the Prison of overprotective pain or anxiety is to live like Truman did before the light fell. We experience our symptoms as structural, as the solid, unmovable, concrete reality of our lives. We feel our heart pounding, our stomach knotting, or our back cramping, and assume it is a report from the live reed of a broken body.

But as we step into this final phase of our journey, our focus moves from the drama on the stage to the mechanics of the theater. We are no longer just trying to survive the production; we are looking for the stagehands.

The secret to rewriting the script is understanding one radical truth: The Warden is not a leader; he is a follower meant to be a Guard that works under our authority. He is a master of surveillance, but he has no eyes of his own. As we discussed at the very beginning of this journey, this is the power of your neuroception—that subconscious security scanner running 24/7 in the background. The Warden doesn't create danger out of thin air; he is simply reacting to what the scanner feeds him. And right now, the scanner is stuck on a loop.

Your Warden is the personification of this system. He relies entirely on the reports coming in from the field. He is constantly eavesdropping on your behavior to see if it's safe to stand down. He is watching your hands, your eyes, and your breath to decide whether to keep the IMAX disaster film running.

This relationship is a two-way street. While the Warden can send a panic signal down to tighten your muscles, your body sends a constant stream of data right back up. In medicine, this internal feedback loop is known as **interoception**, your brain's subconscious perception of your bodily signals.

Ultimately, rewriting the threat script is about retraining these interoceptive pathways. If that data confirms the Warden's fears, the simulation stays active. But if you change the data, you can force him to rewrite the script in favor of reality.

I (Hayley) experienced this firsthand recently while out walking my dogs. Midway through the loop, my hip started to ache when it had been fine for 24 hours. But, I noticed an error in the script: I hadn't been in pain before the walk, and there was no meaningful change in my tissues that would explain a sudden surge in symptoms. That was me catching the stagehands at work.

Instead of bracing against the ache or cutting the walk short, which would have sent danger data right back to my brain, I took a breath and reminded myself that this pain was just an overprotective false alarm. I gently rubbed my leg to interrupt the pain signal with a physical cue of comfort. Because I changed my interpretation, my action followed: I kept walking, and within a few paces, the script rewrote itself. The pain just went away.

The Language of Safety

This is why it is so important to learn the language of safety: it is how you talk back and change the conversation the moment a symptom flares up. When your body sends up an ache or a pang, a dialogue starts.

But your nervous system only speaks two dialects: threat and safety. If you aren't actively changing the topic back to safety when a symptom hits, your brain will naturally continue reading from the script of survival.

When my hip flared up on that walk, and the old threat script started to run, I took on the language of safety by intentionally intervening and actively re-labeling the sensation as a false alarm, thus speaking to the Warden in the only other dialect he understands, safety.

To the Warden, the language of safety is not made of words, but of biological evidence. It is a non-verbal conversation between your behavior and your brain.

While we often use our internal monologue to tell ourselves "it's a false alarm," those words are just the remote control; your body's physical response is the surveillance screen the Warden actually monitors.

That is because the Warden, again, doesn't actually speak English; he speaks biometrics. He doesn't read the thought itself; he measures the physical aftermath of that thought. Constantly checking the tension in your hands, the depth of your breath, and the speed of your movements, the Warden calculates whether your body actually believes your mind.

The Vocabulary: This language is composed of physical cues like soft muscles, rhythmic breathing, and deliberate movement.

The Syntax: It isn't enough to just be calm. You have to provide a consistent stream of data that contradicts the crisis.

The Goal: By learning this language, you aren't just relaxing; you are providing a technical override that forces the Guard/Warden to stand down.

Your brain trusts what you do more than what you think. You can repeat the mantra "everything's ok" a thousand times, but if your jaw is tight and your breath is shallow, the Warden will believe your jaw and breath every single time. He ignores your internal monologue in favor of the physical evidence.

So, to rewrite the script, we have to stop broadcasting the threat signals that keep your Fortress in a state of perpetual lockdown and start identifying the **13 Threat Scripts** unwittingly keeping the Warden convinced that the emergency is still real, and instead learn to speak the language of safety, the only dialect the Warden actually responds to.

Group 1: The Internal Dialogue

The scripts in this category live entirely inside your head, in how you internally narrate your day, interpret your sensations, and handle your emotions.

To the Warden, your thoughts are intelligence data, a live status report from the field. If your thoughts are frantic, hyper-focused on pain, or filled with words of urgency and inadequacy, the Warden assumes the environment is actively threatening. He doesn't see a stressful to-do list or an anxious thought; he sees an emergency, and he keeps the sirens blaring.

To break this cycle, you have to change how you track, describe, and process what is happening inside you.

Threat Script #1 — Constant Monitoring

Waking up and instantly scanning your lower back, head, or stomach like a submarine sonar operator puts your system on immediate patrol. This mimics exactly what ancient man had to do in the truly hostile environment they lived in: watch closely or miss the predator. But in the horror movie of overprotective pain and anxiety, this hyper-vigilance becomes fuel for the fire, because the Warden doesn't care what you find; he only cares that you felt the need to scan in the first place. You don't check your front door locks fourteen times if you live in a world where theft doesn't exist.

The moment you start to monitor your body, your mood, or your environment, you are testifying under oath that the "set" is unsafe. In response, your brain amplifies the signal (making the pain louder and the anxiety sharper) just to help you keep watch.

The Safety Rewrite: Active Indifference

To shatter the simulation, you have to starve the script of the mental and physical reactions it needs to survive. By practicing active indifference, you refuse to feed the fire, effectively cutting off the energy the threat requires to keep running.

Resist the Urge to Investigate: When your imagination starts to run the show, deliberately stop trying to figure the sensation out. Don't try to fight or stop the feeling; simply refuse to analyze it.

Adopt an Indifferent Attitude: Act like a person who is so safe, so bored, and so unbothered by their own internal weather that they don't even bother to check the forecast. Treat the sensation as background noise, not a breaking news headline.

Stop Watching the Screen: Refuse to monitor your body or scan for changes. Treat your physical sensations like a boring television channel you have completely lost interest in. By flatly withholding your focus, you change the station and send a high-level all-clear signal that the Warden cannot ignore.

Threat Script #2 — The Harsh Inner Critic

We often think of our inner critic as a motivational coach, but when you narrate your day with words of urgency ("I'm behind," "I always feel awful," or "I need to fix this right now"), you are providing data of a failing environment. In a survival context, this inadequacy means you are too weak or too slow to survive, so the Warden refuses to let your muscles relax.

The Safety Rewrite: Self-Kindness

To rewrite your inner monologue, replace the critic's harsh corrections with warm self-kindness. When the Warden hears a influential critic screaming in your head, he keeps the sirens blaring. Speaking to yourself with the patience you would offer a dear friend shifts the narrative from a high-stakes thriller to a story of recovery. This kindness isn't just a nice sentiment; it is the strategic biometric evidence your brain needs to know the crisis is over.

Use Third-Person: When your thoughts start to spiral, use your own name (e.g., "Clark is feeling pressured") instead of saying "I." As odd as that might sound, it creates immediate psychological distance, telling your nervous system you are an objective observer of the feed, not the character being crushed by it.

Slow Down Your Inner Monologue: When you notice the internal critic shouting, intentionally repeat the thought in a slow, bored, or even surfer-dude voice. By stripping the catastrophic weight from the tone, you turn a terrifying prophecy into a slow, harmless background noise.

Rename the Situation: Replace "I need to fix this" with "I am tending to this." One is a frantic repair of a failing structure; the other is the steady maintenance of a secure home.

Threat Script #3 — Suppressing Your Emotions

The nervous system views unprocessed emotion as an unsolved variable. In its original design, the ability to push an emotion aside was a survival tool. If you were in the middle of a crisis, you didn't have time to process grief or fear; you had to act. However, your brain expects you to circle back and integrate that feeling once the coast is clear. When you constantly distract yourself or power through, your overprotective brain concludes it still isn't safe to feel, maintaining a high baseline of tension because it thinks you are still on the run.

The Safety Rewrite: Emotional Honesty

To de-escalate the tension, you have to speak the language of emotional honesty in order to prove to your brain that the coast is clear enough to acknowledge your internal world.

Practice the Micro-Check: Instead of distracting yourself the moment a difficult feeling arises, give it thirty seconds of acknowledgment. Naming at least three things you are feeling at the moment (e.g., "I feel frustrated. I feel overwhelmed. And I feel scared") acts as a signal to the Warden that the threat is identified and no longer an invisible variable.

Create Permission Windows: Set aside five minutes where you aren't doing anything. By sitting in stillness without a phone or a task, you demonstrate to your brain that you are in a context where safety is allowed.

Conduct a Behavioral Audit: Instead of trying to force yourself to calm down, ask: "What am I doing right now that suggests I shouldn't calm down yet?" If you are pacing, scrolling rapidly, or jaw-clenching, your brain will trust that behavioral evidence over your desire to be peaceful.

Group 2: The Body Language of Threat

The scripts in this category are all about the physical clues your body is sending up to the Warden.

While we often try to use our internal monologue to tell ourselves "everything is fine," the Warden doesn't actually speak English; he speaks body language. He monitors your physical actions via the vagus nerve, treating your body's tension like a live surveillance screen. If your breathing is shallow, your jaw is clamped, or your grip is heavy, the Warden calculates that your body expects an incoming strike. He will always believe your physical evidence over your mental mantras. To force a standstill, you have to manually change the physical data your body is broadcasting.

Threat Script #4 — Breath-Holding

In a suspense movie, when the killer is in the next room, the protagonist holds their breath to stay silent and small. In the language of safety, breath-holding is the ultimate evidence of a predator being nearby.

In the early 2000s, Linda Stone, a former executive at Apple and Microsoft, realized that the moment she opened her inbox, she stopped breathing. To see if this was a universal instinct, she observed over 200 people, finding that 80% of us succumb to what she later called email apnea; freezing your lungs as if a digital notification were a predator in the brush, telling the Warden, "*Don't let them hear us,*" and keeping your nervous system in high-alert stealth mode.

The Safety Rewrite: Resonant Breathing

You can't feel like you are in a thriller if you are breathing like you're taking a nap. So, in order to rewrite the script, you need to let the Warden take a breath.

Take a Low Belly Sigh: This is your scene transition. When you notice you've been holding your breath, let out a long, audible "Haaaaa"—the sound of someone sinking into a warm bath. This resonant sound is a biological announcement of safety that forces the diaphragm to drop.

Use the Double-Inhale Reset: To physically pop the simulation, take a deep breath in through the nose, and then at the very top, sneak in a second, shorter inhale to maximally inflate the lungs. Then, let out a very long, slow exhale through the mouth.

Threat Script #5 — Vocal Tensing

Your voice is an instant reflection of your nervous system. Under threat, the muscles of your throat instinctively tighten to produce higher-pitched, strained sounds to warn the tribe. To your brain, a tight throat is a clear signal that the action sequence needs to stay active. By tightening the muscles around your larynx, you are physically acting out the script of someone who is being constricted by their environment.

The Safety Rewrite: Vocal Softening

To rewrite the script, you have to change the soundtrack. A thriller won't maintain its tension if the lead actor is calmly humming.

Introduce a Low Hum: Create a resonant, low-frequency hum in your throat. This rhythmic vibration overrides the high-pitched alert signals sent by a stressed vagus nerve.

Trigger a Dramatic Yawn: Intentionally force a wide, deep yawn to physically stretch tight throat muscles and trigger an immediate soft reset of your vocal script.

Lower Your Pitch: Consciously drop the pitch of your voice and soften your throat before speaking to prove to your brain that your voice can afford to take its time.

Threat Script #6 — Physical Guarding

Your nervous system interprets muscle tension as a preparation protocol for impact. From a biological standpoint, guarding was only ever meant to be a temporary state. But, when you live with persistent pain, your system defaults to constant, protective bracing.

The Safety Rewrite: Drop Your Guard

To melt your armor, you have to manually release the protective tensing of your muscles to show the Warden that there is no incoming strike.

Exhale the Struggle: Let out a long, slow breath through your mouth. Your brain monitors your diaphragm more than almost any other muscle; shifting away from short, shallow breaths acts as a biological all-clear signal.

Drop Your Jaw: Practice creating a small space between your upper and lower teeth. When the jaw is soft, the brain finds it nearly impossible to maintain a state of biological stress.

Relax Your Shoulders: Intentionally let your shoulders slump away from your neck, proving to the Warden that you can finally put your shield down.

Threat Script #7 — White-Knuckling

In a thriller, characters always grip the steering wheel or clutch their phones with white knuckles to keep things from slipping away. In overprotective pain, it's easy to hold on for dear life too: stabbing the keyboard keys or trying to crush your smartphone. But in nature, you only grip an object that hard if you are climbing for your life or fighting for a weapon. When you use ten pounds of pressure to hold a four-ounce coffee mug, the Warden assumes the world around that mug is hazardous.

The Safety Rewrite: Drop the Pressure

To rewrite this script, you have to drop the pressure in order to prove to the Warden that the environment is so safe you can afford to be loose with your grip.

Check the Pressure: While typing or driving, check if you could do the task with 50% less force. Practice resting your hands on the wheel instead of strangling it.

Soften Your Grip: Periodically open your palms and wiggle your fingers. Open palms are a universal biological signal that there is nothing left to fight.

Group 3: Rhythms and Routines

The scripts in this category are all about how you spend your time, focus, and your physical surroundings.

In nature, a stable animal moves slowly, focuses deeply on one thing, and maintains steady daily rhythms. Jagged shifts in attention, constant rushing, and erratic schedules only happen when an environment is volatile, like a forest full of predators or a sudden storm.

When you live with a chaotic daily pace, your Warden assumes you are reacting to external emergencies. To settle his fears, you must deliberately show him that the environment is secure enough to allow for steady depth, leisure, and rhythm.

Threat Script #8 — Abrupt Task-Switching (and Self-Interruption)

Your brain's primary job is to predict the near future so it can prepare your body's resources. When you jump-cut between tasks, interrupt your own rest, or switch digital tabs every thirty seconds, you create high unpredictability. Because rapid, jagged shifts in attention only happen during an external crisis, your unstable focus feeds the Warden data suggesting the scene is constantly shifting, forcing him to keep the action sequence running.

The Safety Rewrite: Monotasking Continuity

The way out of this thriller is to provide your brain with consistency. You have to prove to your system that the set is stable enough to stay in one place, effectively boring the Warden into shutting down the action sequence.

Finish One Task: Let one simple task reach its natural end without interruption. Do not let yourself jump-cut to a new screen or project until the current one is put away.

Delay the Pivot: When the sudden urge to switch tasks appears, pause and delay your response for just ten seconds. This short gap breaks your automatic reflex and proves you are in control.

Touch Back Base: If you do get pulled away by an unavoidable interruption, return to your original task briefly before you allow yourself to continue elsewhere to maintain a line of continuity.

Define Your Finish Line: Decide exactly what "done" means before you even begin a task, and intentionally close the loop.

Threat Script #9 — Information Overload

When you spend hours scrolling through feeds, jumping from a tragic news headline to a recipe, then to a notification, you feed the Warden a highly chaotic data stream. Historically, humans only experienced this rapid sensory input when tracking multiple variables in a hostile environment. By doomscrolling, you accidentally mimic a survival scan. The Warden watches your eyes shift every three seconds and assumes you are tracking moving targets, keeping your heart rate up, and cortisol spiked.

The Safety Rewrite: Filter Your Input

To settle an overprotective brain, you have to prove that the world is stable enough to allow for undistracted depth. Closing the tabs and putting down the phone signals to your system that it is safe to be still.

Single-Task Your Focus: Instead of scrolling through ten articles, read one physical book or listen to one long-form podcast. The Warden sees this slow-burn focus as proof that there are no immediate predators to track.

Turn off Notifications: Every notification is a jarring jump-cut in your internal movie. Turn off non-essential pings to tell the Warden the scene is quiet.

Move Your Eyes More Slowly: If you must use your phone, consciously move your eyes slowly. Rapid vertical scrolling mimics a pouncing motion in the wild; slow, horizontal scanning mimics a calm animal grazing.

Threat Script #10 — Unpredictable Rhythms

Historically, humans only ate at random times or slept in fragmented bursts when they were under duress, enduring a famine, or navigating a disaster. When your sleep, meals, and daily structures are completely irregular, you accidentally mimic these survival rhythms. So the Warden decides that your environment is compromised by external dangers that prevent a normal routine, and he refuses to let your nervous system drop into a restorative state.

The Safety Rewrite: Create a Ritual

To reassure your overprotective brain, you have to provide it with repetitive anchors. You don't need a rigid, military schedule, but you do need to prove that your world is stable enough to support a rhythm.

Bookend Your Day: Even if your midday is chaotic, create a simple morning and evening routine that happens at the same time every day. This tells your nervous system that the start and end of your day are secure.

Eat at a Fixed Time: Eat at least one meal a day at a fixed time. The biological signal of a reliable, predictable fuel source is one of the fastest ways to satisfy the Warden's surveillance.

Create a Predictable Transition: Use a specific physical cue, like lighting a candle or changing your clothes, to signal the shift from work to rest. This acts as a visual clapperboard, telling the Warden that the high-stakes scene has officially ended.

Threat Script #11 — Tunnel Vision

Zooming in tight on a single object in a thriller film naturally creates tension. When you're under threat, your vision narrows into a sharp, tunnel-vision stare designed to track a target.

Modern life has us locked into this fixed gaze for eight hours a day on smartphones and laptops, which simulates a prey animal freezing to keep its eyes on a threat. The Warden interprets this unblinking stare as: "*The target is in sight. Do not look away.*"

The Safety Rewrite: Open Your Eyes

To shatter this narrow script, you have to provide the Warden with peripheral data, proving that you are safe enough to relax your focus and scan your wider surroundings.

Use Your Panoramic Vision: Soften your gaze. Without moving your eyes, try to notice the far corners of the room, the space above your monitor, or the wide horizon outside. Engaging this wide-angle view is a physical override that forces your brain to dial down arousal.

Apply the 20-20-20 Rule: Every 20 minutes, look at something 20 feet away for 20 seconds. This simple reset breaks the prey's stare and signals that there is no immediate predator to track.

Threat Script #12 — Hurry

To your nervous system, speed is evidence that you are running out of time and a threat is closing in. In the wild, animals only move at maximum velocity when hunting or escaping danger. Walking rapidly to the bathroom, scarfing down your food, or rushing through a conversation tells the Warden: All this hurry must mean we are escaping something, keeping the hero of the story trapped in a high-speed chase scene.

The Safety Rewrite: Slow Down

To change the script, you must provide the Warden with the pace of peace, proving that you possess the most valuable resource a survival-mode brain can imagine: Time.

Practice the 10% Slow-Down: Intentionally walk, speak, or eat 10% slower than your habit dictates. This slight deceleration acts as a massive all-clear signal to your system.

Breathe an Extra Breath: Before opening a door or starting your car, take one calm, unnecessary breath. This proves to your brain that there is no predator at your heels.

Take a Deliberate Pause: When someone asks you a question, wait two seconds before answering. This peaceful pause tells your brain that the scene is safe enough to allow for thought instead of just reflex.

Threat Script #13 — Avoidance

Your nervous system sees avoidance as absolute validation of danger. If you refuse to do a specific task, like walking to the mailbox or sitting in a certain chair out of fear of pain or a flare-up, the Warden interprets your retreat as a narrow escape from a predator. Of course, sometimes, temporary avoidance is appropriate during an active injury, illness, or flare, but when avoidance becomes a lifestyle rather than a short-term strategy, it reinforces the boundary walls of your prison, confirming to your brain that the avoided area or activity is genuinely hazardous territory. Every time you turn back, the Warden draws the border lines of your life a little smaller, locking you into an ever-shrinking fortress.

The Safety Rewrite: Graded Expansion

To break this cycle, you have to become an evidence gatherer by performing small, calculated experiments to prove the Warden wrong. Reclaiming avoided territory in tiny, non-threatening increments shows your brain that you can handle the scene without a catastrophe occurring.

Shrink the Target: If an activity feels too dangerous to attempt, break it down to a miniature version. Don't walk to the mailbox; just walk to the front door. Don't sit in the "bad" chair for an hour; sit in it for two minutes. Show your brain the first step is secure.

Pair with Comfort: When stepping into an avoided task, intentionally bring a sensory cue of safety with you. Listen to your favorite song, wrap yourself in a warm sweater, or apply the Active Indifference mindset. You are teaching your brain to associate the feared activity with physical comfort.

Celebrate the Attempt, Not the Outcome: Focus entirely on the fact that you crossed the border, regardless of whether a minor symptom flared up. By celebrating the action of showing up, you signal to the Warden that you are an active explorer, not a hiding prey animal.

The Exit Door

Hopefully, it is clear by now that peace isn't a feeling you wait for; it's a conversation you lead, even when all evidence seems to be against you. Identifying these **13 Threat Scripts** is your light fixture moment. It's the first step in moving from being a victim of the live feed to becoming a conscious observer of the mechanics behind the scenes.

The desire to master the language of safety will move you from being a character trapped in a script to the director who decides which scenes are worth keeping. And realizing that the Warden isn't an enemy to be defeated, but a misguided protector who has been reading a faulty script for far too long, should give you a sense of hope.

By systematically starving him of threat data and no longer waiting for the feeling of peace to arrive, you can effectively dismantle the walls of your own prison and make peace inevitable.

Remember, the Warden is meant to be a follower. He is waiting for you to show him what is true. Every time you choose peace over preparation, or leisure over urgency, you are editing the narrative in real-time. The simulation only holds power as long as you believe the painted sky is real.

It's time to stop surviving the production and finally start living the life that exists beyond the set. Take a breath, drop your jaw, and walk through the door.

The coast is clear.

12

Your Inner Pharmacy

The Chemicals of Healing Already Inside You

"The best way out is always through."

— Robert Frost

Today, the siege ends.

For the last eleven chapters, we have been doing the heavy lifting of a restorer. We've mapped the corridors of your overprotective brain, identified the false alarms at the Gatehouse, and started the brave work of rewriting your internal scripts. But even the most skilled restorer needs the right materials to turn a prison back into a fortress.

Up until now, you may have looked for those materials in a bottle, hoping for relief, even if it came with a cost.

But those medications are just pulling levers that are already built into your biology. It's a part of your biology. Your body produces its own pain-relievers, its own calming signals, its own chemistry of safety and connection: Endorphins. Oxytocin. Dopamine. Serotonin. They are part of your design.

External medications can support, amplify, or stabilize this system, but they didn't create it; it belongs to you. That just means that you aren't starting empty. You're starting equipped.

Your system releases these chemicals in response to specific inputs, like movement, safety, connection, meaning, and attention. And it produces them specifically for your body, for free, and available at your fingertips.

Why the Pharmacy Stays Closed

But it does not release them on request. It releases them i**n response to what you do.** And that's exactly where overprotective pain keeps you trapped.

Throughout this journey, we have seen how overprotective pain trains us into a natural, instinctive sequence: FEEL → THINK → DO. We wait to feel safe, assuming that feeling better is the green light required for doing more.

But waiting for overprotective pain to stop before you move is like waiting for your shadow to move out of the way before you step forward; it's not going to happen. If, in overprotective pain, you wait to feel better to change, you will find yourself unable to do more and more until you're trapped so deeply inside your prison that you can't even see the light of day.

Action Must Come Before Feeling: DO → THINK → FEEL

This old instinct is perfectly designed for the Helpful Pain of the flu, a broken ankle, or any situation where your body genuinely needs protection. In those moments of helpful pain, waiting to feel better is how you survive.

But with overprotective pain, the order must flip. We have to lead with the DO, not because we feel like it, but because action is the primary retraining language of the nervous system. By leading with the doing, we stop waiting for fear and pain to give us permission to live. **We move to provide the physical evidence that the level of protection exceeds the actual threat.**

As that evidence builds, the process becomes self-reinforcing. The DO becomes the very trigger that releases the chemistry you've been waiting for—airing out the prison, restoring light, and allowing you to finally begin writing your own prescriptions.

The Proof is in the "Ah-choo"

Whether you know it or not, you've been a practicing pharmacist your entire life; you just haven't been aware of the prescriptions you've been placing. Your internal lab doesn't wait for a doctor's note; it reacts in real-time to the world around you, mixing chemical cocktails that shift your state in seconds.

To jog your memory, just think of the feeling you get when you sneeze. That building tension followed by an explosive "Ah-choo" resets your entire system. That isn't just air moving; it's a targeted drug release.

Or think about how it feels to step into a steaming hot shower on a freezing day. The moment the water hits your skin, you feel a deep, heavy-limbed relaxation spread through your frame. That sigh of your muscles is your pharmacy dosing you with safety signals and heat-activated relaxants.

These are tangible, physical drug releases that prove your pharmacy is constantly at work, responding to every input you give it. In overprotective pain, the pharmacy hasn't stopped working; it has simply been filling the only "prescriptions" it's been receiving; the ones written by an overprotective brain. It has been flooding your system with the chemicals of high alert, waiting for a new kind of order to fill your script.

Your Own Pharmaceutical Lab

This internal lab is your biology's most sophisticated tool for adjusting, regulating, and intervening in your experience of the world. Your body can produce powerful, experience-shaping chemicals, those that ease pain, create calm, deepen connection, and restore balance. These are part of an intelligent system that responds to safety, meaning, movement, and relationship. Many external substances work by interacting with these same systems, sometimes mimicking, sometimes amplifying, sometimes overriding them, but they cannot replicate the precision of your body's own regulation. They simply bypass the system rather than retrain it.

That means relief isn't foreign to you. The pathways already exist.

What your body needs is not more supply, but the right signals. It doesn't release these chemicals indiscriminately. It responds to cues; how you move, what you focus on, whether you feel safe, connected, or threatened. When those signals shift, the system shifts with them.

So the goal is not to replace what medication does, but to understand what your body is already designed to do, and how to work with it. You don't need a new supplier. You need to learn how your system releases what it already knows how to produce.

Endorphins: The Natural Painkiller

Endorphins are among your body's natural opioids, so effective that many of our strongest pain medications were designed to mimic the same opioid receptors they activate. The name endorphin comes from the phrase *endogenous morphine*, coined after scientists discovered that the body produces its own morphine-like compounds. These naturally occurring peptides bind to many of the same receptors targeted by powerful opioid medications, but instead of coming from a pharmacy, they're released by your own body during movement, exertion, stress, social connection, and other meaningful activities.

These drugs are part of an intricate pain-regulation system that adjusts according to context, helping your body decide when pain should be amplified and when it should be quieted.

So it turns out we didn't invent pain relief at all. We just discovered substances that imitate mechanisms the human body was already using.

Writing the Prescription

Your brain produces endorphins through physical demand. They are a survival reward released when your body confronts a specific request for energy or resilience. When you push your physical limit slightly, engage in deep, belly-aching laughter, or even eat spicy food, your brain perceives this demand and releases endorphins to buffer the system. Endorphins are the biological payment for your effort. But if there is no demand, the pharmacy stays closed.

This is why waiting until you are completely out of pain before you start living your life actually backfires; without a demand signal, your brain sees no reason to manufacture the relief you are waiting for. However, creating a demand doesn't mean you have to run a marathon. In 2011, Oxford University researchers discovered that genuine, heavy belly laughter acts as a powerful demand signal for your pharmacy. They proved that just fifteen minutes of social laughter triggers an immediate surge of endorphins, physically expanding a person's pain tolerance by 10 percent without requiring a single ounce of strenuous physical exercise.

How It Works

Once released, these compounds act as your internal volume knob. They bind to opioid receptors throughout your brain and spinal cord, not necessarily to stop every signal, but to dampen the alarm by altering how those signals are interpreted, and stripping away the urgency and weight of the pain. The sensation might still be there, but its urgency and perceived threat have faded, which allows your body to move from protecting to relaxing.

The Comfort Zone Trap

In a state of overprotective pain, your brain is often terrified of any demand. Because it's been taught that even small efforts are dangerous, you avoid the very inputs that trigger an endorphin release. But by staying within your safe zone of total comfort, without even realizing it, you have inadvertently kept the pharmacy doors locked. By not placing the physical demand on your body, you deprive your brain of the exact biological trigger it needs to justify unlocking your internal medicine dispensary.

The Silent Soldier

When I (Hayley) think of how much power the brain has over pain, I think of my father-in-law, who, during WWII, was hiding with his platoon behind enemy lines in the dense jungles of Burma. His platoon had dug in for the night, covering their "shallow graves" with grass and brush to hide from the enemy. As a Japanese patrol moved through the clearing where they had dug in, the enemy had spread out and was randomly plunging bayonets into the ground to find anyone hiding, when one of those bayonets went straight through my father-in-law's shoulder.

Biting down on a stick, he didn't make a sound. He didn't flinch. He just stayed pinned to the earth, silent, until the bayonet was lifted and the footsteps faded away. It wasn't until much later, when the patrol had passed, that he actually felt the full pain of the wound.

That is the perfect example of your brain's extraordinary ability to regulate pain. His brain recognized that a scream would be a death sentence for him and his platoon, so it instantly muted the signal. It didn't stop the injury; it just turned down the alarm long enough for him to survive. Scientists now know that this kind of pain suppression can involve powerful internal pain-relief systems, including the body's own opioid-like chemicals.

And you live with the same survival machine. Right now, it might be keeping your volume turned up because it thinks that's the safest move, but the story in Burma proves that your brain *can* change that volume in a heartbeat if it just believes there's a better way to protect you. So we aren't asking you to ignore your pain; we're letting you know that your brain can find a reason to turn the volume down.

Dopamine: The Engine Starter

If endorphins are about blocking the bad, dopamine is about providing the good. While it is often simplified as the pleasure chemical, its role in your pharmacy is much more strategic than that: it is the chemical of motivation, anticipation, and pursuit; the biological "Yes" that makes an action feel worth taking.

Think of dopamine as your brain's internal fuel for the hunt, designed to keep you moving toward things that help you survive: food, water, connection, and safety. Dopamine provides the electric spark of focus and energy that allows you to start the journey towards those things. That is because **dopamine is the primary tool used to shift from a state of "I can't" to a state of "I'm doing it"** by sharpening your vision, alerting your nervous system, and turning a daunting task into a series of reachable goals.

How It Works

Once released, dopamine floods the prefrontal cortex to provide the chemical go-signal that makes effort feel possible in the first place. This aligns with Dr. Wolfram Schultz's pioneering work on **Reward Prediction Error.** In it, he discovered that dopamine doesn't actually fire when you receive a reward; it fires during the *anticipation* of it. It is the chemical of the chase, designed to fuel your forward momentum before you ever cross the finish line.

By rewarding even the anticipation of success, it pulls you out of stagnation and provides the physical momentum needed to override the guarding of your overprotective brain.

Writing the Prescription

Your brain produces dopamine through prediction and pursuit. It's released when your brain anticipates a win or achieves a goal. But not all dopamine is created equal. You can get some cheap dopamine in passive spikes from things like scrolling social media or eating sugar, but these are quick hits that leave you feeling empty and stunted afterward.

This is where a lot of us accidentally short-circuit our own recovery. When you are trapped on the couch, miserable and hurting, your brain is starved for a win. Naturally, you reach for the closest comfort available: scrolling through social media, binge-watching TV, or eating a sugary snack. These activities trigger a quick, passive spike of dopamine that feels like a temporary relief, but it is what we call **cheap dopamine.**

Because these modern spikes are so unnaturally intense, your brain sees them as a dangerous overload. And your nervous system, which is obsessed with balance, in an attempt to protect its delicate circuits from literally frying from overstimulation, deploys a defense mechanism: by dynamically down-regulating, or closing down, its own dopamine receptors. Essentially, it puts in earplugs to survive the noise.

Unfortunately, the next day, you wake up in a biochemical deficit. With half your receptors closed for business, ordinary life suddenly feels dull, and your baseline motivation flatlines. Because your natural drive is gone, the overprotective alarms in your brain feel louder and more intense than ever, and you're left looking for an external hit to jump-start your motivation.

The Tragedy of Dopamine Collapse

When you wake up in this biochemical deficit, your overprotective brain fundamentally changes its scanning settings. It completely stops looking for wins and starts looking exclusively for threats. Because your brain is convinced you are under a permanent state of siege, it pulls the plug on your forward momentum. It redirects your entire metabolic budget away from exploration, joy, and movement, using it instead to fund the heavy production costs of its internal horror movie.

As your dopamine reserves bottom out, you don't just feel physically tired; your brain's internal engine completely stalls. Without this vital chemical currency to accurately measure effort, your brain suddenly labels even tiny, safe movements as an impossible mountain that isn't worth the energy.

This biochemical bankruptcy is what locks the cage of fear-based avoidance. What feels to you like a total loss of willpower is actually just a motivational engine that has been completely drained of its gas.

The Lost Keys

I (Hayley) know exactly how terrifying it is to live with a bankrupt pharmacy, because for years, I was the one with the empty medicine cabinet.

After living under the crushing weight of overprotective stress and being on high alert for every single twinge, pop, and ache in my body, my world started to shrink. Out of fear, I stopped doing the things I loved. I stopped socializing, stopped moving, and started withdrawing. Before I knew it, I had become almost a complete shut-in.

At a time when I should have been full of life, I felt twenty years my senior. My joints were stiff, my muscles were constantly sore, and I was plagued by unrelenting migraines. My nervous system was so fragile and hyper-vigilant that I developed severe food sensitivities to almost everything I ate. I felt completely trapped inside a body that had become a prison.

What I didn't realize at the time was that because I was trapped in the FEEL → THINK → DO cycle, I was constantly waiting to feel safe, comfortable, or energetic before I dared to live my life. And because that comfort never came, I never placed the order to my pharmacy. Then my brain just looked at my isolation and immobility and assumed we were under a permanent siege, so it kept filling the same script: more stress hormones, more vigilance, and more pain.

My turnaround happened when I finally found the door to my inner pharmacy and realized all I had to do was access it, to stop waiting for permission from my pain to do that, and to manually override the system. Even while stiff, sore, and terrified, I had to do what I didn't want to do: start moving before I felt better. With that, I started manufacturing micro-wins, leaning into tiny moments/doses of connection, and celebrating small physical victories. In short, I started writing my own prescriptions.

Slowly but surely, the pharmacy started filling my prescriptions. As the dopamine, endorphins, oxytocin, and serotonin started to flood back into a system that had been starved for years, my life opened back up. The migraines receded, the food sensitivities quieted down, and the stiffness melted away. I didn't just get my health back, I got back all of my vim, vigor, and vitality.

I want to tell you now, you are not a broken machine waiting for an external mechanic. You have a fully-stocked pharmacy. You just need to learn how to sign the script.

The Supply Line

To re-open this vital supply line, you just have to change the currency you're using. In this pharmacy, the only currency your brain accepts is physical action, if only walking to the mailbox or doing two minutes of stretching. This is what it takes to pay the upfront cost of effort before you feel like it.

While you can't think your way into a dopamine surge, you can force your brain to manufacture it by changing the data it receives. Every time you choose physical action over avoidance, you override the system. When you invest in an earned victory, however small, your brain adapts by opening more receptors over time. By consistently funding these expensive micro-wins, you literally increase your psychological credit limit, making the next day's movement feel easier, lighter, and completely within your budget.

But your motivational engine isn't the only system the Warden can hijack. While dopamine provides the drive to pursue life, your inner pharmacy houses an equally powerful chemical designed to do something entirely different: neutralize your fear.

Oxytocin: The Safety Signal

Next, we have oxytocin, the ultimate neutralizer of the stress response. In your internal lab, it acts like the most potent anti-anxiety medication available. While it is often nicknamed the cuddle hormone, its role in recovery is much more clinical: it is the biological signal for safety and trust, the chemical all-clear that tells your nervous system it no longer needs to maintain a defensive posture. When oxytocin is present, your brain's fear center (the amygdala) is physically dampened, allowing your body to shift out of survival mode and into repair mode.

Writing the Prescription

The prescription for oxytocin comes through connection and co-regulation; generated when your nervous system feels felt or supported by another. And it goes beyond physical touch to eye contact, shared laughter, a deep conversation, or even the presence of a trusted pet. It's the chemical byproduct of belonging. And when you experience a moment of genuine connection, your brain perceives that you are not alone in the hunt, and it releases oxytocin as a biological insurance policy against stress.

How It Works

Once released, oxytocin acts like your internal system neutralizer. It travels through the bloodstream to lower your blood pressure and reduce the production of cortisol (the stress hormone), not just making you feel warm and fuzzy, but physically altering the state of your nervous system by increasing your vagal tone, your body's ability to move from high-stress guarding back into a state of calm. This is the chemical bridge that allows your muscles to finally let go and your heart rate to steady.

The Proof

We touched on her research earlier, but in 2009, Dr. Naomi Eisenberger and her colleague Sarah Master at UCLA conducted another experiment that perfectly illustrates how oxytocin acts as a stress neutralizer. In the experiment, they asked women in committed relationships to undergo controlled heat pain on their forearms under several different conditions. In some rounds, the women held a squeeze ball. In others, they held the hand of a total stranger. But in the key rounds, they either held their partner's hand or just looked at a photograph of him.

The results were stunning. When the women held their partner's hand, their pain ratings dropped significantly. But the bonus was that looking at a photograph of their partner worked just as well, and in some cases, even better, than the physical touch.

Oddly, when they held a stranger's hand, the pain actually felt worse. The presence of a stranger was a threat signal that dialed the volume up. But the reminder of a trusted relationship shifted the system out of threat and into safety. It engaged the brain's pain-regulation pathways and released a prescription for safety chemicals. Their bodies responded accordingly, not by eliminating the heat, but by decreasing its intensity and urgency.

The Lesson for Your Recovery

In overprotective pain, it is this signaling that has been lost. Naturally, because pain is isolating, we can stop sending our nervous system cues of safety and connection, resulting in a state of high-alert vigilance where we stop looking at the photos of safety and start imagining the images of threat.

To pull your system out of this lockdown, your recovery demands that you manually feed these safety cues back into your life. By intentionally rebuilding small bridges of connection, you force the amygdala to stand down, re-enlisting oxytocin to start dampening the alarms from the inside out.

The Isolation Tax

The real tax of this isolation isn't just loneliness; it's a state of chemical vulnerability. When you let your world shrink to the size of a couch, you're effectively leaving the gates of your nervous system completely unguarded.

To stop paying this tax, you have to actively override the urge to hide. You can't treat connection as a *luxury* you get to enjoy after you heal; you have to treat it as the active medication required to jump-start the process.

The Supply Line

We aren't just talking about being social. We are talking about a biological override for your alarm system. By intentionally seeking out moments of connection and co-regulation, you are airing out the fortress from the inside out and flooding your system with the one chemical that tells your brain it is finally safe to stop the siege.

Serotonin: The Mood Stabilizer

If endorphins block the pain and dopamine drives the pursuit, Serotonin is the chemical that sustains the peace. In your inner pharmacy, it acts as your ultimate mood stabilizer and emotional anchor. While it's often associated with general happiness, its clinical role in recovery is all about status, safety, and self-efficacy. Meaning, it's the chemical signal that tells your brain, "*You are capable, you are in control, and you belong.*" When serotonin levels are healthy, your nervous system is resilient, meaning you can handle minor physical or emotional stressors without instantly locking down into a defensive posture.

Writing the Prescription

Perhaps surprisingly, your brain produces serotonin through reflection, pride, and, believe it or not, sunlight. So it's triggered when you acknowledge your own progress, practice gratitude, or remember a time you felt powerful and capable. This is why rewriting your internal scripts is so important. When you shift from viewing yourself as a broken patient to a capable restorer, your brain physically rewards that shift in status with a dose of serotonin. It's also highly responsive to basic biological rhythms, like getting morning sunlight into your eyes and moving your body outdoors.

The Alpha Experiment

The role serotonin plays as your system's baseline stabilizer becomes clear in a series of groundbreaking behavioral studies conducted on primates. Researchers tracked the internal chemistry of alpha males, the leaders of the pack who enjoyed the highest status, the safest territory, and the total respect of their community. When an animal was in this secure, dominant position, its serotonin levels were sky-high. They moved with calm confidence, rarely overreacting to minor disturbances.

But then, the researchers introduced a twist. They separated the alpha male from his pack using a one-way mirror, allowing him to see his community but preventing them from seeing or responding to his leadership cues. Isolated and ignored, his perceived status plummeted.

Within days, his serotonin levels crashed. The physical and behavioral transformation was staggering: the once-calm leader became anxious, submissive, and violently hypersensitive to the slightest threats in his environment. But when researchers artificially restored his serotonin, his anxiety vanished, and his calm composure returned.

This is the exact loop at play in your recovery. Overprotective pain is a master at demoting your internal status. It makes you feel isolated, submissive to your symptoms, and completely stripped of your agency, which causes your serotonin to tank. When your serotonin drops, your nervous system loses its baseline shield. It becomes raw and brittle, interpreting even a minor, safe physical sensation as a catastrophic emergency.

How It Works

Once released, serotonin acts as a heavy-duty background filter regulating your daily threshold for threat. When serotonin levels are healthy, your system possesses a thick layer of chemical insulation, meaning it can easily filter out minor physical or emotional stressors spiraling into a catastrophic overreaction.

But when you are trapped in a lockdown of overprotective pain, that insulation wears thin. And without enough serotonin to filter out the background static, your threshold drops to zero. That means if a tiny whisper of sensory data is allowed to pass through the gates completely unedited, your system will treat it like a major explosion.

That's because serotonin works closely with your brain's emotional center to prevent catastrophic thinking. It keeps you grounded, ensuring that a small flare-up doesn't turn into an emotional tailspin, keeping your system steady enough to stay in the DO → THINK → FEEL sequence.

The Lost Agency

In a state of overprotective pain, your serotonin lines are constantly depleted because the Warden strips away your sense of control. When you feel powerless against your body and your internal agency drops, your brain literally halts serotonin production. It concludes that because you are no longer in command, you shouldn't waste resources on stabilizing your mood or filtering your data.

This chemical shutdown is what leaves your nervous system completely raw and highly susceptible to those false alarms. You aren't fragile because you lack willpower; you are fragile because your brain has paused the manufacturing of its primary stabilizer.

The Supply Line

Like the rest of your internal drugs, you can't just force a serotonin surge, but you can build it brick by brick. By celebrating tiny victories, tracking your daily progress, and intentionally practicing gratitude for what your body can do, you send a clear message to your brain: I am winning. That shift in perspective forces the inner pharmacy to reopen the serotonin tap, stabilizing your nervous system and giving you the emotional bedrock needed to take back your fortress.

The Placebo: A Prescription from the Mind

For decades, we've treated the placebo effect like a trick played on a weak mind, a way to prove to researchers that a medicine works. But in your inner lab, the placebo effect is the single greatest proof that your pharmacy is working.

The magic isn't actually in the capsule; it's in the expectation. The moment you believe relief is on the way, your brain essentially signs its own prescription pad. Because it's been told exactly what that little pill is supposed to do, it anticipates a win and immediately starts prepping your body for comfort. So when someone swallows a sugar pill, and their pain vanishes, it's not a trick or "all in their head"—their brain has literally just flooded their system with a real, physical dose of its own home-brewed dopamine and endorphins.

The Naloxone Proof

In a famous study, dental researchers gave patients a placebo for pain. As expected, many felt better. But then, the researchers secretly administered Naloxone, a medication used in emergency rooms to block the effects of opioids.

The result? The placebo relief vanished instantly, and the pain came rushing back.

Unfortunately for these participants, this proved once and for all that the relief wasn't just a mind trick; it was driven by real, physical chemistry. The brain had literally manufactured its own internal narcotics, and Naloxone came in and flipped the switch off. Naloxone didn't block a placebo effect in their minds; it blocked the physical endorphins their brain had just flooded into their system.

This changes everything because it means the placebo effect isn't a psychological illusion or a trick of the mind, but a physical command to prescribe a real chemical. Their brains didn't just imagine feeling better; they quite literally wrote a prescription, went to the shelf, and manufactured their own morphine. Their minds thought, and their bodies did.

It's like that moment in The Matrix when Morpheus points out that if you get hurt in the simulation, you bleed in the real world because "*the mind makes it real.*" Inside your inner pharmacy, that isn't just movie sci-fi. It's a literal biological fact.

Changing the Order

These powerful painkillers in your inner pharmacy are already sitting on the shelves, fully stocked and ready to go. But as we've seen, they require a signature on the prescription pad before they can be released.

For years, you might have been waiting for the feeling of safety, comfort, or confidence to arrive before you take action. But your inner pharmacy doesn't work backward. If you want the chemistry of relief, you can't just wait for fear and pain to give you permission to move. You have to sign the script yourself.

In the next chapter, we are going to walk straight into your biological parole hearing, where you are going to get the Six Keys required to manually override your brain's defensive posture and unlock your inner pharmacy's deepest vault of natural relief. The drugs are ready—it's time to learn how to place the order.

13

Placing the Order

Six Keys to Unlocking Your Inner Pharmacy

"It is not because things are difficult that we do not dare; it is because we do not dare that they are difficult."
— Seneca

Imagine walking downhill. The slope is steep, and every ounce of your momentum wants to pull you downward. Which means that you don't really have to work at going that way because the gravity of the terrain does most of the work for you. It's easy to just let your feet fly, lean into the incline, and descend into the valley because it requires almost no effort at all.

In mathematics, this is the Markov Chain, which describes a system that naturally drifts downhill toward the path of least resistance. On a surface with hills and valleys, the most likely state is always the bottom of the deepest valley. Which means that a system, whether it's a set of numbers or a human nervous system, will naturally settle into the deepest valley because it requires the least amount of energy to stay there.

For years, the downhill direction for your overprotective brain has been a maximum security lockdown. After years of high alert, your nervous system has found it easier to just assume the worst than to investigate and measure the truth. It triggers the sirens not because there is an intruder, but because that deep valley of protection is the most practiced, energy-efficient response it knows. Which means that it has become your biological default.

You can think of this overprotection as a rut in the road created by a heavy wagon traveling the same muddy path for a decade. Eventually, the ruts become so deep that the wheels find them automatically. You don't have to choose to brace your shoulders, hold your breath, or trigger a flare. The wheels of your nervous system just drop into the groove of guarding because that is where they have spent the most time. This is the downhill path of the overprotective brain. It's the tendency for your nervous system to choose the heavy, guarded, and painful path because it has become the most familiar track on the map.

But you don't have to stay in this rut of overprotection. You are not a permanent resident of this lockdown. You can get out of the groove and start the climb toward something better by reawakening the parts of yourself that have become dormant from years of protection. Even with the gravity of a thousand past lockdowns pulling at you, the slope only influences where you tend to go; it doesn't remove your power to move from a prison to a fortress.

The Parole Hearing

To move from a prison of overprotection back to a Fortress requires a parole hearing.

In a traditional prison, a parole board doesn't just look at the crime that put you there; they look at your behavior while incarcerated. They are looking for evidence of rehabilitation. Your Warden is doing the same thing. He's watching how you handle your day-to-day life inside the lockdown of overprotective pain. If you are constantly tensing for impact or avoiding movement, the Warden sees that as evidence that the world is still a dangerous place.

To win your parole, you have to stop speaking the Warden's default language of **FEEL → THINK → DO** (FEEL a spike, THINK you're in danger, DO nothing). Instead, you must force a manual override using the action-first script of **DO → THINK → FEEL:**

DO: Initiate an intentional safety signal that contradicts a lockdown (a movement, a breath, a change of scenery). You aren't waiting for the pain to stop; you are performing an act of rehabilitative behavior.

THINK: Certify to the brain that the action is safe. If you move but your mind is screaming, "This is going to kill me," the Warden stays in lockdown. Your conscious thought provides the Warden with the legal cover he needs to change the standing order.

FEEL: The Warden's verdict. When he sees the DO and the THINK match up without a catastrophe, he authorizes a chemical release, flooding your corridors with the exact home-brewed chemistry needed for that moment.

This sequence is how you fill out the prescription. Now, let's look at the raw ingredients you have available. **We call these the Six Keys to Unlocking Your Inner Pharmacy.**

Placing the order

You have your operating system in the DO → THINK → FEEL cycle—but every prescription needs the right active ingredients to actually work. That's where the Six Keys to Unlocking Your Inner Pharmacy come in. Think of these as the specific instructions for authorizing a refill. When you use them, you're providing the Warden with undeniable proof that the lockdown is unnecessary, finally allowing him to dispense the pharmacy's most powerful relief.

Key #1: Sub-Maximal Aerobic Movement (The Endorphin Pump)

In a healthy body, movement acts like a pump that naturally distributes pain-relieving chemicals from your inner pharmacy to your tissues. But when you've been trapped in the pain cycle for a long time, that pump gets rusty and locks up. To get those chemicals flowing again, you have to trick the Warden into letting the supply through.

And you do that with one simple rule: Uninterrupted, easy movement.

Sub-maximal aerobic movement is anything you do continually that keeps your effort well below your absolute limit. **Here's your golden rule**: You have to be able to carry on a full conversation without gasping for breath. If you are breathing too heavily to talk to a friend next to you, you've gone too far. You've crossed the line into a hard workout, which the Warden will immediately view as a threat, and he will shut the pharmacy doors flat.

Think of gentle, steady rhythm over intensity. We're talking about an easy walk around the neighborhood, a relaxed swim, or a light ride on a stationary bike. This is not the time for running, a high-intensity aerobics class, or anything that leaves you dripping in sweat and huffing for air.

Note: If you have a strenuous job, like a nurse logging 20,000 steps a shift, you are moving, but biologically, it doesn't activate the pharmacy. That's because stressful, chaotic work steps keep your brain on high alert. To trigger your inner pharmacy, your movement must be peaceful, intentional, and entirely separate from your job.

The Prescription

To get that peaceful, intentional movement, you need a specific plan. Endorphins are your body's built-in pain-relief system, but after long periods of high alert, that system becomes incredibly hard to access. To re-engage it, you have to carefully dose your activity so you don't trigger the system's defenses.

How to Prime the Pump

When your body has been stuck on high alert for months or years, your brain is hyper-focused on protecting you. So, the minute you start moving, your brain's immediate reaction is going to be to scream, "Stop!"

But as you keep moving, you start to change the data your brain is receiving.

Around the twenty-minute mark of continuous, easy movement, your brain finally gets enough data to realize, "Oh, wait. We can do this. The situation isn't as dangerous as we predicted."

That is the exact moment the brain signs off on a fresh prescription. Endorphins and other natural painkillers start flooding your bloodstream. It doesn't happen like a sudden jolt of caffeine; it feels more like a slow, warming wave. But the sharp edge of your pain starts to dull, your muscles stop tensing up for impact, and your body finally switches out of panic mode.

Micro-Movements (The Calibration)

Now, look: if you are trapped deep in the Prison right now, reading the words "twenty minutes of continuous movement" might sound like we're asking you to climb Mount Everest. We aren't. What I (Sam) ask my clients is to start small, with micro-movements. Micro-movements are tiny, bite-sized doses of activity designed to prove to the Warden that movement is safe, without triggering a flare-up.

That means you sit on a stationary bike with zero resistance and pedal for just three minutes to start, then you're done. Or, maybe you just walk around your house for a few minutes, or stretch on a yoga mat.

Just do your three minutes on day one. If your system handles it without panicking, try four minutes on day three. Then five. What we are doing is slowly building a tolerance, laying down the tracks so that eventually, you can hit that twenty-minute mark where the real chemistry floods in. We just need to meet your body where it is today, not where you want it to be next month.

I once worked with a woman who felt like she couldn't even do something as simple as walking her dog. To her overprotective brain, the sidewalk was a minefield.

So I asked her to just clip the leash to her dog's collar and walk twenty feet to the edge of the driveway and back.

She later told me that this was the hardest thing she'd ever done. But by just making that tiny move, she was performing a calibration and sending a safety signal that proved to her Warden that the world hadn't ended and her body hadn't broken.

By keeping these shifts small enough to stay under the radar, we aren't just exercising; we are performing tiny surgical strikes that prove that hurt is not equal to harm. This calibration allows our brains to return to normal function and finally authorize the release of our internal medication.

Key #2: Hobbies and Meaningful Engagement (The Joy Trigger)

Your inner pharmacy doesn't just respond to movement; it responds to meaning. In the Prison, survival is your only assignment, so the Warden locks down anything that isn't directly tied to keeping you alive. Creativity, curiosity, and play are treated as luxury items you can't afford. Over time, your hobbies disappear, interests fade, and the things you used to love start to feel totally pointless.

But when you immerse yourself in something mildly enjoyable, absorbing, or purposeful, you stage a prison break. You flip the switch on your brain's reward system, sending a wave of dopamine and natural calming chemicals through your body. This chemistry pulls your nervous system out of panic mode and reminds your brain that it is safe to turn the pain volume down.

Stress Breakers vs. Stress Makers

So, what counts as a "Joy Trigger"? It isn't about achievement; it's about engagement.

- *Good examples*: Working on a puzzle, knitting, painting, gardening, or reading a gripping novel.
- *The Video Game Trap:* Gaming can work if it absorbs your attention, but use caution. If you are playing for hours just to numb out and escape reality, it stops having a positive impact.
- *The Sports Trap:* If you choose a sport, ask yourself: How competitive is it? If a casual game of pickup basketball turns into an angry, high-stakes battle, it becomes a stress maker, not a stress breaker.

The Prescription

Start small. Set a timer for 5–10 minutes and choose one activity that holds your attention just enough to keep you there. Your only goal is to stay engaged for the full time. Each time you do this, the Warden adjusts, and the pharmacy is given another prescription to fill.

Key #3: Strategic Relaxation (The System Reset)

If the Warden is in a constant state of lockdown, it's because he is sensing a threat based on the data coming from your body. When your breathing is shallow, and your muscles are tense, you are sending a high-priority alert to your brain that says: "*Predators are on my heels and I've got to run*." And as long as the Warden hears that signal, he will refuse to open the Pharmacy for anything other than survival chemicals.

Strategic relaxation is the key that unlocks your pharmacy's primary natural sedative: gamma-aminobutyric acid, or GABA.

The "Predator" Signal vs. The GABA Prescription

The Warden won't authorize the release of this calming agent if he thinks you are seconds away from being caught. And without relaxation, your body stays in a high-voltage state that keeps the GABA bottle on the shelf.

By intentionally slowing your respiratory rate and softening your muscles, you are writing a prescription that lowers your sense of danger by showing the Warden that if you were truly being hunted, you wouldn't be able to breathe this deeply or sit this still. Once he sees that evidence, the prescription goes through for the Pharmacy to flood the corridors with GABA, which physically dissolves the tension of the lockdown.

The Busy Intersection Rule

The most common mistake a pharmacist makes is trying to write this prescription for the first time while the sirens are screaming. If you wait until a massive pain flare hits to try belly breathing, the Warden will be too panicked to fill the prescription.

Relaxation is a skill, not a rescue flare. Imagine trying to learn how to ride a bicycle for the first time while crossing a busy, six-lane intersection during rush hour. You'll crash, and your brain will decide that bikes are dangerous. That means that to make this key work, you have to practice it in a quiet, sunlit driveway, when you already feel safe, until the muscle memory of relaxation is so strong that you can trigger it even when the world gets loud.

The Prescription

To unlock the GABA and Serotonin required to activate your night maintenance crew, you have to use tools that provide the Warden with undeniable proof of safety:

Diaphragmatic Breathing: Focusing on the belly to physically stimulate the Vagus nerve. This is the direct hotline to the Pharmacy that says, "The predator is gone. Switch to rest and repair mode."

Sensory Buffers: Using me-time or noise-canceling headphones to give the Warden a break from the constant noise of the world.

Rhythmic Stillness: Activities like rowing, paddleboarding, or even rhythmic breathing. The steady, predictable pattern provides the Warden with a prescription to follow, allowing the physical bracing to dissolve so the GABA can do its work.

By building this skill in the quiet of your life, you are teaching your nervous system that it has the capacity to dial back the intensity. You are proving to the Warden that peace isn't just a lucky break, it's a prescription that you have the power to write.

Key #4: Laughter (The Emotional Override)

While it is easy to write laughter off as fluffy or unnecessary, it is actually one of the fastest ways to change your body's chemistry. Famously, the historic monthly *Reader's Digest* published, "Laughter is the best medicine" and they weren't far off.

Biologically, it is nearly impossible for negative emotions and stress chemistry to remain active when you laugh. Laughter is an instant pattern-interrupter. It sends an undeniable safety signal straight to the Warden's desk, forcing your body to drop cortisol levels and release endorphins. It doesn't erase the pain, but it immediately changes the state in which your brain processes it.

Since your brain prioritizes any evidence that contradicts a threat, laughter is the fastest way to hand-deliver that testimony to his desk.

The Prescription

Frequency matters more than intensity. Short, repeated moments of authentic laughter throughout the day have a greater impact than waiting for a single, larger release. Your body doesn't need spontaneity to write the prescription; even intentional laughter can deliver endorphins into your system.

Laughter does not solve the problem; it just changes the state in which the problem is processed. And when the state changes, the Inner Pharmacy is given room to respond with chemistry that supports regulation rather than protection.

Key #5 Positive Social Interactions

Isolation removes one of the strongest signals the brain uses to assess safety. Without it, the system has fewer reasons to reduce protection, and your Inner Pharmacy remains aligned with vigilance, instead of regulation. But positive social interaction changes that signal.

Connection tells the brain something it cannot generate on its own: that you are not alone, and that the environment is stable enough to engage. The presence of another person, especially one perceived as safe, alters how your nervous system allocates its resources.

The shift builds through repeated, tolerable experiences, and these moments provide evidence that engagement does not require the same level of defense.

The Safety Signal

In your Inner Pharmacy, Oxytocin is prescribed when you engage in meaningful connection, whether it's a shared laugh with a coworker, a deep conversation with a friend, or even a brief, positive exchange at a coffee shop. You are filling a high-priority prescription.

Oxytocin tells your system: "*I am not alone, and this environment is safe enough to engage.*" In the presence of Oxytocin, your brain's emergency-only orders are overruled, and the Pharmacy stops flooding your body with isolation-fueled stress chemicals and starts releasing the compounds that allow you to feel grounded and secure.

Reclaiming the Lost Territory

For many of us in lockdown, the world has become a series of no-go zones where you lose your seat at the Friday night dinner table, your spot on the team, and your role in the office because the Warden tells you that staying away is the only way to stay safe.

But every time you step back into those spaces, you are submitting evidence at your Parole Hearing and are proving that the world is not a predator-filled wasteland. As the Warden learns that you can survive uncontrolled environments, you reclaim activities you thought you'd never experience again and you go from prisoner to resident while the Warden returns to his valued role of Guard.

By building the skill of connection, starting in small, safe doses, your parole comes through, and you move from Prison to Fortress, proving that the Pharmacy's best stabilizers aren't found in a bottle, but in the deliberate choice to stop hiding and start engaging.

The Prescription

In the Pharmacy, the purity of the drug is more important than the size of the pill. Your brain is far more influenced by the depth of an interaction than the number of people you see. Well-being peaks at roughly 2 to 6 face-to-face interactions per day, adding more people doesn't add more Oxytocin.

If your lockdown baseline is zero, do not try to force casual socializing. Start safely:

Enlist a professional: Book a session with a coach, counselor, or physical therapist. This guarantees a safe, structured, and deeply meaningful interaction.

Pick one safe person: Schedule a brief coffee or phone call with just one trusted friend who understands your situation.

Aim for two meaningful encounters per week as you work up to more.

Key #6: Food

Important Note: If you have a history of diagnosed or undiagnosed eating disorders or disordered eating, please skip this section. Your journey requires a specialized approach; defer to your clinical team instead.

If the first five keys are about getting the Warden to sign the orders and the Pharmacist to dispense the meds, Key #6 is about keeping the lab stocked with raw materials. Nutrition isn't a drug itself, but it is the infrastructure support for every chemical reaction in your body.

Think of it this way: the most brilliant Pharmacist in the world cannot fulfill a prescription if the shelves in the back are empty. Proper fuel affects your chemistry availability; that chemistry affects how your system regulates itself; and that regulation is what ultimately determines whether the volume on your pain is turned up or down.

Food as Infrastructure

We often hear food is fuel, which is true, but it's also lumber, copper wiring, and concrete. Your body is constantly under renovation. To build a resilient Fortress, the Lab needs a steady delivery of diverse resources.

In our Pharmacy, no food group is bad or illegal. Carbs, fats, and proteins are simply different types of inventory. Carbohydrates are the high-octane energy the lab needs to keep the lights on. Proteins are the building blocks used to repair the pipes and wiring. Fats are essential for protecting the nerves and maintaining the integrity of the Pharmacy walls.

Restrictive dieting or moralizing food (labeling things "good" vs. "evil") only stresses the system, which alerts the Warden. We aren't looking for a diet plan; we are looking for Infrastructure Support.

The Chemistry of Regulation

You already know the basics: more whole foods, more fruits and vegetables, less processed baggage, and less alcohol. But here is why it matters for your Pharmacy:

When you provide the Lab with high-quality resources, your faculties can perform at their highest level. Poor fuel leads to noisy chemistry. If the Lab is trying to create stabilizers like GABA or endorphins using low-grade materials, the results will be poorer outcomes. On the other hand, a well-nourished system is a regulated system. When the body has the resources it needs, the Warden doesn't have to panic over resource scarcity, allowing the system to shift from a state of emergency to a state of high-performance maintenance.

The Prescription

To keep the Lab running at peak capacity, your stocking order should focus on availability rather than restriction:

Whole Food Delivery: Prioritize foods in their natural state to give the Pharmacist the complex micronutrients needed to compound your internal meds.

Diverse Inventory: Eat a wide variety of colors. Different resources provide different chemical building blocks.

Reliable Logistics: Feed the system regularly to prevent blood sugar crashes that the Warden misinterprets as a biological threat.

Minimize Poisons: Avoid artificial preservatives, flavors, colors, and sweeteners (like nitrates, aspartame, or sucralose). These chemical additives tip off the alarms and set an already hyper-sensitive immune system on high alert.

Nourishing the Lab ensures that when you use your other keys, the Pharmacy actually has the raw ingredients on hand to fulfill the order.

Rebuilding the Council Chamber

None of these Six Keys represents the path of least resistance. It's always easier to stay on the couch than to walk for twenty minutes, and it is easier to isolate in the dark than to find a reason to laugh. In the Prison of overprotective pain, the easiest path to temporary safety is avoidance.

Avoidance is the Warden's favorite tool. He whispers that the only way to stay safe is to do less, see fewer people, and move as little as possible, until your world shrinks to the size of a postage stamp.

To break this cycle, you have to re-enter the Council Chamber, the leadership center of your brain that weighs consequences and makes deliberate choices, because in a system stuck in lockdown, the Council has lost its gavel since the Warden has been shouting urgent commands for so long. But when you choose to do the hard thing anyway, you perform a manual override, walking into that dusty Council Chamber, striking the desk with the gavel, and physically strengthening your prefrontal cortex through top-down regulation. Finally, you are telling the alarm system, *"I hear the sirens, but we are moving anyway."*

In the gym of the fortress, resisting avoidance is the heavy weight we all have to lift. Real biological change doesn't happen when a task feels pleasant; it happens in the exact moment you push back against the urge to do nothing.

But here is a crucial ray of hope as you lift this weight: regression to the mean. That simply means that in biology, extremes always balance out over time. A massive flare-up or a terrible day is a temporary statistical outlier, not your permanent reality. That's because your system naturally wants to return to a stable baseline, and pushing through the initial resistance helps your body find that healing balance faster.

Real biological change happens in the exact moment you push back against the urge to do nothing. But to understand just how tightly the Warden has restricted your Council's view, you have to look at the conditions of your release.

The Conditions of Release

In Emma Donoghue's 2010 novel *Room*, inspired by harrowing real-life events, a young woman named Joy Newsome (Ma) and her five-year-old son, Jack, live in a 12x12-foot soundproof shed. Their entire world is contained in that space: a bed, a toilet, a tub, a rudimentary kitchen, and a television. While the TV shows them glimpses of a world beyond, the only physical connection to the outside is a single skylight cut into the ceiling.

This is the only world Jack knows. Ma has raised him to believe that only the things inside *Room* are real. While he sees trees, animals, and other people on the screen, he believes they are just images in outer space, unreachable and make-believe. What holds him there is not just the lock on the door, but the story he has been given about what is real and what is dangerous.

That is how an overprotective brain works. When your system has been focused on threat for long enough, that becomes your world: the pain, the discomfort, and the ever-increasing limits that start to define you. The Warden, like Ma, convinces your system that what you feel is the full territory.

The turning point in *Room* was not a change in their physical circumstances; it was a change in what Jack believed. When he finally realized the world on the television was real, the Warden's power started to crumble, because the same system that defines the limits of your world also controls the state of your body.

The Action of Safety

Your Inner Pharmacy cannot operate in a state of captivity. It won't release the good stuff if the Warden is still convinced a zombie is at the door. You aren't going to fix your situation by decorating the interior rooms or trying to make the pain slightly more comfortable.

The actions you take today, the laughter, the movement, the stubborn refusal to believe the Warden's latest special report, are you rolling yourself into the rug. It is you playing dead to the old story so you can be carried out into the light.

It feels risky, we know, like your system is lying to you, but the same biology that defined the limits of your world is the same biology that can expand them. You aren't fighting for a better prison; you are retraining your system to recognize that the door was never actually locked, and that the prison was really a fortress all along.

The Warden's Final Stand

But here is a warning for a body seeking parole: When you start to push for freedom, the Warden will most likely get louder.

In *Room*, when Jack finally tries to escape, it is terrifying. He has to roll himself in a rug, play dead, and trust that the outside won't kill him. To his nervous system, the escape was more dangerous than the captivity.

When you start using these Six Keys, your Warden is going to panic. He's going to see you moving, breathing, and engaging, and he's going to scream that you are making a mistake. You might experience a temporary flare, a spike in alarm, or even an increase in symptoms as your system tests the new boundaries. In the Prison, you would have interpreted this as proof that you are broken.

In the Fortress, it's time to recognize this for what it is: The Warden's last-ditch effort to pull you back into the interior rooms. Just as the sun hurt Jack's eyes the first time he saw the sky, your new freedom might feel overwhelming as the old narrative is being challenged.

The Shift to Abundance

Think of this as a structural renovation. You don't have to rebuild the entire Fortress in an hour; you don't even need to place a daily order with your internal pharmacy. But every time you engage a key, you are producing a chemical safety signal that replaces a brick of fear with a brick of resilience and retraining your system to recognize that the door was never actually locked, and that the prison was really a fortress all along.

As you repeatedly experience safety in the places where the Warden predicted threat, your biology actually changes. The Editor in your prefrontal cortex regains his grip, the

Sergeant at the Gatehouse starts to muffle the noise, and the zombies lose their power to paralyze you.

You are not a victim trapped in a cell; you are a resident who has discovered the door was never actually locked. The Warden is no longer your master, but a Guard who must learn to stand down, and the Zombies are merely the echoes of an exhausted, overprotective system. Using the Six Keys is undeniably more demanding than the strategies of the past, but it is the only way to move from a life of survival to a life of abundance.

The keys are in your hands. Your parole is being processed. It's time to move out of the interior rooms, stop managed survival, and start manufactured freedom.

The door is open. The pharmacy is yours. Get up, walk out, and don't look back.

14

The Chemistry of Safety

The Overprotective Brain Reset

"It is not the mountain we conquer, but ourselves."

— Sir Edmund Hillary

In the 1994 film The Shawshank Redemption, the elderly Brooks Hatlen, portrayed by Morgan Freeman, is finally paroled after fifty years behind bars. He is handed a cheap suit, escorted through the heavy iron gates, and given a room in a boarding house. By every physical measure, the state has declared him a free man.

Trouble is, Brooks' nervous system never got the message.

When he sits on the city bus, his eyes dart wildly, and his trembling hands fearfully grip the frame of the seat, physically terrified by the roaring speed of a world that moved past him decades ago.

At his new job, bagging groceries, he can't even use the restroom without first asking a manager for permission. The prison walls are gone, but every action, breath, and micro-movement proves he is still locked inside, still a prisoner to a mind organized entirely around confinement.

Institutionalized by his time in prison, Brooks became so deeply adapted to the rigid rules of confinement that freedom actually felt like a threat to him.

Ironically, that same institutionalization that kept Brooks a prisoner after being set free is the pathology of the overprotective brain.

When you live with an overprotective system for months or even years, you don't just have pain; you become institutionalized by it. Your survival instincts become your personality.

To reverse those instincts, we have to navigate what criminologists call re-entry. For a prisoner, re-entry isn't just about walking out the front gate; it involves the grueling work of learning how to be yourself again. Re-entry requires making a choice without asking permission and walking down a street without constantly scanning for danger.

It's the process of deconditioning: a systematic re-wiring of a nervous system that has become a professional survivor. We decondition by intentionally:

1. Disrupting the rules of the cell and breaking old protocols

2. Reclaiming your agency from the grip of your symptoms

3. Flooding your hyper-focused, defensive brain with the sensory novelty of the outside world.

This process of re-entry is the only way to resolve the core biological conflict of your overprotective symptoms. You can't just will yourself to be better, because you are up against a fundamental law of human chemistry, which states that the chemistry of safety cannot flourish in a system still organized around danger.

The Chemistry of Danger vs. The Chemistry of Safety

The reason re-entry feels so much like a battle lies in your inner broadcast. This is what biologists call **The Displacement Effect**: your nervous system is physically incapable of prioritizing two conflicting signals at the same time.

An institutionalized nervous system becomes locked onto a danger frequency—a high-volume broadcast of cortisol, adrenaline, hyper-vigilance, and prediction scanning. Because the brain prioritizes survival signals above all else, restorative chemistry struggles to break through the noise.

Which basically means that your brain is so busy shouting "Stay Alert!" it literally can't hear the pharmacy door opening.

If the Six Keys from Chapter 12 are the *tools* to unlock your healing, the internal broadcast is the environment where you use them. You can have the best keys in the world, but if the door is buried behind a ten-foot wall of white noise, you won't even find the lock.

Your Inner Pharmacy is fully stocked, but vigilance keeps *Danger Radio* playing on repeat. Vigilance acts as a biological lockout. You can't feel the soothing effects of your own restorative chemistry while your body is still acting like it's behind bars. So, to open the door, we don't need more medicine; we just need to change the broadcast.

The Priority of Survival

Why is *Danger Radio* so loud? Because your brain is a survival machine, not a joy machine. And to a brain built for survival, a 1% chance of threat can sometimes matter more than a 99% chance of joy. Because if you miss an opportunity for joy, you're disappointed. But if you miss a threat, you're dead.

This is why joy becomes so hard to access when you are in pain. Your brain isn't refusing to be happy; it's prioritizing survival. In other words, defense can consume so much of your biological bandwidth that there is less available for restoration. Helping your nervous system de-escalate the threat frees up more of that bandwidth for recovery and healing.

Imagine your mind as a high-stakes control room. Joy is fantastic for day-to-day operations, but she has a low security clearance. The moment your system detects even a whisper of a threat, an emergency protocol takes over, and the entire hierarchy shifts instantly.

In the Pixar film *Inside Out*, the character of Fear lives for these exact moments. The second a potential hazard appears on screen, he doesn't wait for consensus; he just pushes Joy away from the console, takes the levers himself, and hits the panic button. It's a total operational takeover, wherein the biological signals for peace and repair are locked out until the alarm stops ringing.

And your brain learns from these repeated internal conditions. If you spend all day scanning for pain and bracing your muscles, you are essentially training your brain to stay on a danger frequency. Over time, that frequency becomes your baseline. And this is how a prison is built: through the repetition of survival.

The Chemistry of Danger

When your nervous system becomes institutionalized this way, your brain is essentially a chemical production plant locked into a danger contract. To keep you alive in what it perceives as a high-stakes environment, the plant runs 24/7, flooding your bloodstream with cortisol and adrenaline. These aren't bad chemicals; their design is flawless, their timing is just off, prioritizing immediate survival over long-term repair. In the wild, adrenaline and cortisol spike for 10 minutes to help you outrun a predator, and then they drop back to zero so the safety chemistry can repair the wear and tear.

But inside this internal institution, your brain scans for pain, senses a threat, and keeps the order forms for cortisol and adrenaline signed 24/7. Of course, you don't want to eliminate your danger chemistry; you need it. You just want to stop the plant from running the emergency shift when you are trying to rest.

The trouble is that under this relentless danger broadcast, your body enters a state of sympathetic dominance. As your attention narrows to a laser focus on potential threats, your brain initiates a process called prediction scanning. Simultaneously, your muscles pre-contract into a rigid layer of muscular guarding, turning your body into a suit of armor while inflammatory activation ramps up to prepare for potential injury. In this high-voltage state, your brain shifts its resources away from repair and restoration and toward defense. This is the baseline of the cell, a system expertly designed to endure, but entirely unable to rest.

The precise mechanics of this breakdown are well-documented in motor-control research as "**The Centipede Effect,**" named after the old nineteenth-century poem where a malicious toad asks a centipede exactly how it manages to coordinate all one hundred of its legs. The centipede stops, tries to consciously calculate the precise sequence of its footsteps, and becomes so utterly overwhelmed by tracking its own data that it trips over itself and lies distracted and paralyzed in a ditch.

In sports science, researchers see this exact phenomenon when elite athletes choke under pressure. When an expert golfer or basketball player gets anxious, they stop trusting their automatic, fluid nervous system and start hyper-focusing on the micro-movements of their wrists or the precise angle of their elbows. The moment they bring conscious surveillance to a deeply automated biological system, the fluid mechanics collapse, the physical muscles stiffen, and they miss the shot completely.

When your system is institutionalized by overprotective symptoms, your brain does the same thing to your internal biology. By obsessively tracking heart rate variability, monitoring digestion, or checking how a joint feels after every single movement, you are forcing your conscious mind to micromanage your autonomic nervous system. You are trying to manually coordinate the centipede's legs, and it is exhausting your body.

Your body can be completely still, but if your mind is still pacing back and forth in the watchtower, the doors to the Inner Pharmacy are going to stay locked. To get the healing broadcast of *Safety Radio* to flow, you have to do the one thing that feels the most terrifying to an institutionalized brain: you have to stand down. You have to step away from the spotlight, lower the binoculars, and give your nervous system the only evidence it actually trusts—the total silence of your attention.

The precise antidote to this psychological trap shows up in Harry Potter lore. To summon a protective Patronus shield against the joy-sucking Dementors, a wizard has to focus all their thoughts on a happy memory. Crucially, the shield only stands as long as his attention stays on that memory. The moment he panics, shifting his focus away from the memory to monitor the Dementor's movements and brace for impact, his protective barrier instantly collapses. Just like in real life, the mere act of hyper-focusing on the threat ensures the magic fades, and the alarm keeps ringing.

Fortunately, biology is a two-way street. Just as your nervous system learns to adapt to a lifetime of institutionalized threat, it can train itself to inhabit a reality of safety. By intentionally wielding the Six Keys to your Inner Pharmacy from Chapter 12, even in small doses, you hand-deliver the physical evidence your brain needs to realize the prison gates are open. Systematically rewriting the chemical baseline of your existence overrides the survival machinery and allows the restorative broadcast of *Safety Radio* to finally reclaim the console.

The Chemistry of Safety

By contrast, the Chemistry of Safety is restorative. This chemistry is powered by endorphins, oxytocin, and dopamine, chemicals that don't just feel good, but actually signal to your body to begin the work of repair.

When you shift into this frequency, you enter parasympathetic ease. Here, the biological lockout is lifted. Your muscles soften, your breath deepens, and your focus expands from threat to possibility. And note, this is the only state in which restorative healing can occur: the place where creativity, social engagement, and exploratory behavior live. Essentially, in the chemistry of safety, your brain finally moves from being a professional survivor to an active participant in life.

The Divided System

But moving into this frequency requires crossing a massive, yawning gap. You can use the Six Keys to your Inner Pharmacy perfectly, but if your behavioral power supply is still pumping out danger, your system stays stuck.

This happens because your brain doesn't actually care about what you know; it only cares about what you do. You can tell yourself "I'm safe" a thousand times a day, but if you are still mentally checking your body to see how you feel, your brain assumes you are in trouble. To your overprotective brain, the act of searching for pain is definitive proof that pain is a threat. It's like constantly looking over your shoulder to see if you're being followed. When you do that, your brain stays convinced a predator is on your heels.

What you are experiencing is a glitch in your internal alarm system, a loop that operates exactly like a compulsive habit, feeding on itself without your awareness. When your nervous system becomes institutionalized by overprotective symptoms, your brain starts treating totally ordinary sensations (a mild ache, a quick twinge, a dull throb) as code-red threats. You find yourself trapped in a cycle of constant policing: checking, analyzing, tensing up, or looking for reassurance just to regain a tiny sense of control.

The tragedy of these protective rituals is their hidden cost: every time you mentally or physically engage with the threat to keep yourself safe, you unintentionally reinforce your brain's belief that danger is present. This is why the needle doesn't move. The ritual that gives you five minutes of psychological relief signs a twenty-four-hour extension on the threat response. **Your system just can't heal while your mind is actively treating your body like a crime scene.**

Breaking the Loop

Why do these somatic compulsions have such a hypnotic hold?

Because they work, at least for a moment.

Imagine you're at a restaurant or a friend's house, and you realize the only available seat is "the wrong chair." Instantly, your brain flashes a warning: *"If I sit here, I'm going to get a migraine."* Your anxiety spikes. Even if you sit down, you aren't actually present anymore. Your body may be in the chair, but your mind is running a full diagnostic scan, checking your vision for blurry spots, or tensing your neck muscles to brace for the coming attack.

You might even find yourself constantly adjusting your posture and looking for an exit, just in case.

In that moment, if you move to a different chair or keep obsessively checking your symptoms, your anxiety drops because you feel like you've mitigated the risk. But your brain looks at that sequence and learns a devastating lesson: The only reason we didn't get a migraine (or survived the one we got) is because we stayed on high alert. By performing the ritual, the tensing up, the scanning, the chair-checking, you only validate your brain's initial panic.

To help your overprotective brain stand down, we can borrow a powerful principle from OCD treatment called **Exposure and Response Prevention (ERP)**, which is to say, learning the terrifying art of feeling a sensation, recognizing that the alarm may exceed the actual threat, and choosing not to deploy the compulsion.

Simple as that. Of course, it's not as simple as that, but yet it is.

All that is required is that you let your anxiety peak and fall on its own while you continue doing the dishes or watching the movie, thus giving your system the only evidence it actually trusts: the fact that you turned off the flashlight, stepped away from the ritual, and the world didn't end.

The Identity of Fragility

This kind of constant hyper-vigilance isn't just a bad habit; it eventually shapes who you think you are.

Your nervous system is not an objective machine that just records data and reads it like a cold robot. It's an active listener, constantly eavesdropping on the narrative you tell yourself about your body. If your inner story is that you are fragile, broken, or one "wrong chair" away from disaster, your brain reads that identity as a blueprint for danger.

Institutionalized by overprotective symptoms for years, pain stops being something you simply experience and becomes who you are.

This identity shows up in those repetitive scripts you run in your head every single day without even realizing it. Statements like:

"I am just a sick person."

"My body is completely hypersensitive."

"I just can't handle stress like other people."

Every time you repeat these phrases, your brain reads them as architectural blueprints. It looks at your narrative and says, "*Got it. We are fragile. So, we have to stay on high alert to protect ourselves.*" In response, your nervous system predicts vulnerability, keeping your muscles tight, your nerves sensitive, and your alarm system alarming.

Without realizing it, you have fallen into a neurological phenomenon popularized by some of our most famous cinematic stories: **Stockholm Syndrome.**

Think of the psychological arc of a character like Harley Quinn inside Arkham Asylum. Initially terrified of her captor, the prolonged isolation and inescapable threat cause her mind to undergo a radical, defensive shift. Instead of fighting her captors, her brain decides that her highest probability of survival comes from aligning with them. So, she stops trying to escape, falls in love with the madman running the prison, and actively starts defending the very person who locked her away.

When your overprotective symptoms last for years, your nervous system can initiate this same kind of distorted survival loop in which your conscious mind unconsciously bonds with its captor, the Warden. Rationalizing why you have to stay inside, making excuses for your overactive alarm system, and fiercely defending your own limitations, you become the primary protector of your own prison.

To an embattled brain, inhabiting the predictable role of a sick person feels infinitely safer than risking the chaotic uncertainty of trying to be whole again. You are standing outside your own cell, armed with a rifle, guarding the Warden who locked you in.

And yet, this fierce defense of the cage isn't born out of some kind of weakness; it's driven by a terrifying, unvoiced question: *"Who am I without my illness?"*

When a baseline of pain or exhaustion has dictated every choice, relationship, and boundary for a decade, shedding that identity feels less like healing and more like an existential vertigo. If you're suddenly well, the entire ecosystem of your life shifts overnight. How will your partner interact with you when you no longer need saving? What will you talk about with friends when your symptoms are no longer the central topic of conversation? What will you do with your days when you can no longer blame the biological lockdown for unfulfilled potential?

To change your identity is to mourn the familiar version of yourself, even the miserable version, and step into a vacuum. Facing the known constraints of a sick person takes endurance, but facing the blank canvas of health takes profound, terrifying courage.

The Shift Toward Safety

Stepping away from that familiar cell door means fundamentally changing how you interact with your body every morning. Up until now, your daily life has likely been an exhausting war against your own skin. You wake up, scan the horizon, and immediately stand against your threats. In that rigid pattern, your entire existence has shrunk down to a single, hyper-focused question: *How much do I hurt right now?*

Whether your pain sits at a 2, a 5, or a flat-out 10, on a scale of 1 to 10, the biological truth remains the same. If you are waiting for that number to hit a perfect zero before you allow yourself to participate in your own life, you will remain trapped in a holding pattern indefinitely. By letting a single digit dictate your entire existence, you are accidentally blocking the exact healing you are working so hard to construct.

The truth is that healing isn't just about eliminating symptoms. Of course, we want them gone, but physiological recovery can only begin when you actively increase your system's access to the chemistry of safety.

None of this implies your symptoms are a fabrication; they are real, physical experiences generated by a survival system that doesn't give up easily. Helpful Pain and Overprotective Pain often coexist. The goal isn't to ignore your body's signals, but to stop organizing your entire life around them.

You are not fragile. You are adaptive. Your nervous system simply learned protection through relentless repetition, and because it learned it, it is entirely capable of learning safety.

True healing is the deliberate process of teaching your body that it's allowed to inhabit the world again, even while the background noise is still humming. To break out of captivity, you have to start looking beyond the perimeter of your cell and actively dismantle the bars, one daily decision at a time.

The Warden's Final Strategy

On your journey toward freedom, you are likely to encounter one last, highly seductive trap: turning healing itself into an extension of the prison.

Because your brain is still operating from a place of fear, it will attempt to treat your new health routines the way it treats your symptoms, as things that must be controlled at all costs.

At first, this might look like progress. You add supplements, clean up your diet, and track your sleep. And suddenly you're feeling responsible, proactive, and empowered. Then, because this rigid structure temporarily calms your anxiety, it gives the illusion that you are getting better.

But look closer, and you'll see that the old survival program has just hijacked your new habits. And slowly, these healing strategies become institutionalized.

The problem isn't the healthy behaviors themselves. The problem is that your life has just been reorganized around a new set of fears. You aren't just scanning your body for symptoms; now you're hyper-vigilantly scanning your environment to protect the new routine you built to prevent them.

Without realizing it, the rules can start multiplying:

Don't miss the supplements.

Don't mess with the routine.

Don't stay up too late.

Don't overdo it.

Don't eat the wrong thing.

Don't miss the walk.

Don't skip the protocol.

And just like before, your body is living one mistake away from collapse.

It's still a prison, but the walls are cleaner, the language is more medical, and your routines are healthier, but your life is still being organized around the same thing as before: preventing danger.

Without realizing it, you've traded one cell for another. Think of it as a neurological bait-and-switch straight out of The Matrix. Drinking the green juice and tracking your heart rate variability makes it feel like you've finally escaped the system, when in reality, the Warden has just upgraded you to a more comfortable simulation. Like Cypher, who chose to plug back into a digital illusion because the real world was too unpredictable, your brain clings to the rigid control of a hyper-regulated routine. True, messy freedom feels like too much of a threat. And so over time, your nervous system starts believing that perfect regulation is what stands between you and catastrophe.

Rebuilding the Council Chamber

To break out of this hyper-regulated simulation, your Council Chamber has to issue a final executive order.

Remember, the Warden's favorite trick is to keep your leadership center so terrified of a flare-up that it willingly micromanages your entire life. But the moment you choose to step out into the world anyway, before your routines are perfect, or while a symptom is still humming, the Council officially reclaims its gavel. You aren't trying to quiet the alarms; you are simply refusing to let them dictate your coordinates.

When the Warden has hijacked your healthy routines—turning your diet, your supplements, and your bedtime into an inflexible steel cage—the Council cannot restore safety by thinking harder. It has to act defiantly. To strip the Warden of his authority, the Council must pass three non-negotiable statutes of behavioral sovereignty:

Executive Order 1: *The Principle of Deliberate Imperfection*

If your routine dictates that you must sleep exactly eight hours, drink green juice by 8:00 AM, and take six supplements or face a catastrophic flare-up, you must intentionally introduce tactical variance. Drink a coffee instead. Sleep for seven hours and go about your day anyway. Prove to your brain that your biology is a resilient ecosystem, not a fragile glass sculpture that shatters at the first missed step.

Executive Order 2: *Strip the Warden's Veto Power*

The Warden's primary tool is the threat of an impending symptom used to cancel plans. The Council's counter-order is simple: we do not alter coordinates based on an alarm. If a friend invites you out, and the Warden flashes a warning about the restaurant's lighting or the drive home, you go anyway. You accept that a flare-up is possible, but you decide that living a restricted life in a gilded cage is a far worse consequence than temporary physical discomfort.

Executive Order 3: *Revoke the Micro-Check*

The Council must officially ban the manual tracking of automated systems. You must take off the fitness tracker for a week. Stop charting your symptoms on an app. Stop assessing your digestion after every bite. By cutting off the Warden's data supply, you starve the threat-detection system of the fuel it needs to keep *Danger Radio* on the air.

Implementing these orders might feel terrifying because you aren't just changing your schedule; you are actively dismantling the protective perimeter you built to survive. For months or years, those rigid routines were the only boundaries keeping your anxiety at bay. When you step outside of them, your brain doesn't just feel unprotected; it feels like it is stepping off the edge of the known earth.

This is the ultimate illusion of the overprotective brain: it convinces you that the tiny, highly regulated perimeter of your routine is the only place where survival is possible. To understand the sheer scale of the psychological matrix your Council is finally pushing past, you have to look at the unique conditions of your release.

To understand the sheer scale of the illusion your Council is finally pushing past, you have to look at how easily an overprotective environment can rewrite your entire definition of reality.

The Conditions of Release

Remember, in Emma Donoghue's novel *Room*, a young woman and her five-year-old son, Jack, live captive in a 12x12-foot soundproof shed. Their entire world is contained in that space: a bed, a toilet, a tub, and a television. While the TV shows them glimpses of a world beyond, Jack has been raised to believe that only the things inside Room are real. He believes trees, animals, and other people on the screen are just unreachable make-believe.

What holds him there is not just the lock on the door, but the story he has been given about what is real and what is dangerous.

That is exactly how an overprotective brain works. When your system has been focused on threat for long enough, your limitations become your entire world. The Warden convinces your Council Chamber that what you feel inside the cell is the full extent of the territory. The turning point for Jack was not an immediate change in his physical environment; it was a change in what he believed. The moment he realized the outside world was real, the Warden's illusion crumbled.

Living As Though The Threat Has Passed

When you depend on a rigid routine to feel safe, your life inevitably becomes a high-stakes waiting game. You find yourself constantly pausing at the door, refusing to step out into the world until your environment is controlled and your symptoms are perfectly quiet.

But here is the key: **if you wait for total silence from your nervous system before you start living again, you will be waiting forever.** The very act of waiting for the perfect moment is just another form of scanning, a lingering hesitation that tells your brain there is still a threat outside, keeping your internal power supply firmly set to Danger.

Breaking out of this prison requires a profound shift in strategy: you must learn to live as though the threat has passed.

Now, please understand, this is not an act of reckless denial. This is not about forcing your body through a grueling workout while screaming at yourself to ignore the agony, nor is it about pretending your symptoms don't exist while toughing it out. That isn't safety; that's just another war.

Instead, the answer begins by recognizing the war for what it really is: a life increasingly organized around fear.

Without even realizing it, you have allowed fear to hold the veto power over every decision you make. Your calendar is no longer a reflection of your true desires; it has become a tactical, defensive map designed to avoid a biological landmine. You are no longer living a life; you are managing a threat.

When you decisively choose to live as though the threat has passed, you officially resign from your position as the coordinator of chaos. You stand down.

Does that mean the pain just vanishes? No. Absolutely not.

Standing down doesn't mean you magically feel perfect on day one. Instead, it means that when a sharp twinge suddenly appears, or when the dark shadow of a migraine creeps into the periphery of your awareness, you do not alter your trajectory. Although your instincts scream at you to retreat, you do not change your plans. You do not run for cover. Courageously, you look directly at the sensation, acknowledge its presence like an uninvited guest at a party, and you keep moving anyway.

You choose to let the symptom throw its frantic tantrum in the backseat while you keep your hands firmly on the steering wheel, driving purposefully toward the things that bring you joy.

15

The Fortress Restored

Reclaiming Movement, Identity, and Life

"The only way to find out what is influenced by circumstance is to try to do the thing you think you cannot do."

— Frances Hodgson Burnett

In the heart of Rome stands the Castel Sant'Angelo; a towering stone fortress built on the banks of the Tiber River. It was originally commissioned by Emperor Hadrian as a magnificent, peaceful sanctuary known as the Mausoleum. It was designed to be a place of beauty, reverence, and quiet reflection, open to the bright Italian sky and lined with grand marble statues.

But as the Roman Empire started to fracture and waves of violent foreign invaders swept through the valleys, the city fell into chaos, and the peaceful monument was forced to adapt in order to survive.

Out of absolute necessity, the citizens transformed the sanctuary into an impenetrable fortress. They bricked over the beautiful, open archways to create solid, unyielding defensive walls. They literally dismantled the grand marble facings and tore down the magnificent statues, dragging them up to the ramparts to throw down as projectiles against attackers. The peaceful sanctuary was encased in a grim, heavy, fortified shell.

For centuries, it served its new purpose as Rome's ultimate refuge. When a crisis struck, popes and citizens would flee down a secret, fortified corridor to find shelter within its walls. Protection was embedded into its very design. But long after those medieval wars ended, the structure remained locked in its militarized state, a heavy, closed-off stronghold out of step with the peaceful world growing around it. Its defensive adaptations had become a permanent, rigid fixture.

It took deliberate, courageous labor by master restorers to return the structure to the people. But they didn't do it by tearing down the historic walls, nor denying its past. Instead, they cleared out the debris of old conflicts, opened the blocked pathways, unbricked the windows, and turned the grim stronghold into a place of historical beauty, filled with public life.

Today, the heavy fortifications are nothing but historic exhibits, and visitors walk freely through sun-drenched courtyards flooded with light. The fortress, finally restored to its true intent, is now a place where life can safely unfold.

Your Fortress, Restored

This book has been the story of your own Castel Sant'Angelo, and this is the exact work required to reclaim your own fortress. Your body was never intended to be a battlefield or prison. It was built to be a sanctuary, a place where your life could unfold without tension, urgency, or constant surveillance.

When the human system is running on its original programming, protection operates entirely in the background. Your nervous system silently manages a massive, subterranean economy, balancing blood flow, regulating chemistry, and interpreting billions of safe data points per second, without ever requiring a conscious thought from you.

But when overprotective pain takes hold, it alters the very architecture of your life. Under the prolonged stress of perceived threat, your brain acts exactly like those desperate Roman citizens, sacrificing its finest assets to build a reinforced wall. It bricks up your vulnerabilities for "support." It takes your movement, your vitality, your social connection, and your joy, those statues that made your life magnificent, and smashes them to use as structural barriers against the world.

The Warden puts the fortress into a state of permanent panic, treating the normal friction of everyday living like an invading horde.

But the work of this book has not been to tear down your system's defensive walls, or to smash the alarms. Your alarm system is a marvel of biological engineering, a brilliant, highly sophisticated mechanism designed to keep you safe.

Instead, this process is much closer to the work of a master historical restorer. When an expert approaches a darkened, centuries-old monument, they don't tear down the structure. They meticulously clear away the thick, accumulated layers of carbon, soot, and grime that have built up over years of exposure and trauma. Underneath that heavy film, the original, pristine masonry is still perfectly intact, waiting to be revealed.

Your original design is still there as well. You don't need to rewrite your entire biology or undergo some kind of aggressive, painful medical overhaul to force your body back into submission. But by shifting the order from FEELING to DOING, you can dissolve the overprotective layers of fear and excess protection that have obscured your vitality.

For your fortress, we are talking about doing the architectural labor of unbricking the windows, clearing out the old trauma, and forcing the overprotective Warden to stand down. Rejoining life means realizing that you hold the key to the front gates. You don't have to wait for the Warden to fully fall silent, or for the fortress to feel completely quiet. You are allowed to turn the lock, throw open the gates, walk out into the valley, and live your life before certainty fully arrives.

But this does require a radical shift in your identity. For too long, the Warden has forced your attention inward, demanding that you obsessively track every microscopic sensation, every dull ache, and every potential flare-up. True restoration requires widening your attention outward again. You have to stop feeling the need to micro-manage your heartbeat, audit your breathing, and cross-examine every safe physical movement for hidden dangers. And you must learn to just inhabit the space.

Leading with action allows you to welcome life back into the courtyard where uninhibited movement starts to feel good as you stretch, bend, and interact with the physical world, treating your body like a vehicle for experience instead of a fragile pathology to be constantly audited. As you look beyond the walls, you will start to find your why again, the work, the hobbies, the callings, and the daily contributions that give your life weight and significance.

In this new order, engaging in creative expression forces your brain to dedicate its neural bandwidth to something far more complex and beautiful than a survival loop, giving your mind a better story to tell.

And you do not need a written guarantee from your body that you will be entirely pain-free before you choose this path. You take it because you are alive today, and that's enough.

The Ultimate Paradox

This brings us to the ultimate, uncompromising paradox of your recovery. The grand prescription of this book possibly requires you to do the exact thing you have spent months or years avoiding, and the exact thing your brain is screaming at you not to do: live.

Think back to the Introduction and Colin Craven in *The Secret Garden*. Earlier, we looked at how a corrupted belief system kept him bedridden, paralyzed by the mere expectation of illness. But there is a second, far more agonizing half to Colin's liberation that we must confront now.

Colin's healing wasn't accomplished with a painless flash of insight but with friction. The first time he tried to stand on his own two feet, his muscles screamed, his heart raced, and every protective instinct he had begged him to lie back down. He did not want to stand. It felt too dangerous, too exhausting, and utterly counterintuitive.

What cured Colin wasn't the magic of the garden; it was his own defiance. He broke the prison of his room because he chose to endure the terrifying discomfort of doing the very thing he was convinced would break him.

The prescription for your own life carries that same weight. It requires you to do what, up until now, you could not do, did not want to do, and absolutely do not want to do today.

Whether your remaining symptoms reflect Helpful Pain, Overprotective Pain, or some combination of the two, waiting for them to vanish before you step back into the world is an elegant trap. It keeps you a permanent resident of the fortress, pacing the dark corridors, waiting for a permission slip that your biology is too terrified to sign.

The inner workings of the prison are not dismantled by a change in your symptoms; they are dismantled by a change in your behavior. When you choose to step out into the sun anyway, when you pick up the paintbrush, sit at the dinner table with friends, or walk down the driveway while the Warden is still shouting from the ramparts, you change the power dynamic entirely. You stop asking the fortress for safety, and you start commanding it. You do not break the prison by fighting the walls. You dissolve the prison by outgrowing it.

The Warden's Last Stand

As you walk out of these gates, you have to now prepare yourself for the inevitable: the Warden will not stand down without a fight. The moment you decide to take a walk, accept a social invitation, or lean into an old hobby, your brain's old alarm system will likely flare. In psychology, this is sometimes called an **extinction burst.** When an old protective pattern begins losing its influence, it often makes one final, dramatic attempt to regain control screaming that you are making a mistake. Trying to use the familiar sensations of pain and panic to force you back into the dark corridors where it believes it can keep you safe.

Expect the pushback, and do not assume that a flare-up automatically means new damage.

When the alarm sounds in the middle of your new life, the worst thing you could do is to run back inside the fortress. Instead, pause, take a breath, and recognize the flare-up for what it truly is: the frantic, desperate pacing of an old guard who hasn't realized the war is over. Look the Warden in the eye and keep moving.

Millimeter by Millimeter

Remember, too, that the master restorers didn't transform Castel Sant'Angelo overnight. They cleared the debris stone by stone. They dissolve the dark varnish millimeter by millimeter.

In the same way, don't demand an instant transformation from your body. Recovery is a cumulative economy. Every single time you choose action over avoidance, you are removing an old barrier, clearing off old varnish, and teaching your brain a new language, the language of capability, strength, and presence.

The walls of your biological sanctuary took time to encase you, and they will take time to open. Trust the masonry of consistency.

Step Into the Light

The blueprint is in your hands. The keys are in the lock. The pharmacy is open.

You no longer have to spend your days surviving a production of fear, auditing your biology, and treating your own skin like a cage. The sky above you is real, the valley is waiting, and the coast is entirely clear.

You have spent long enough guarding your fortress; now it's time to step out into the sun, drop your jaw, breathe the open air, and finally reclaim your life.

Open the gates. Your sanctuary awaits.

About the authors

Dr. Sam Tyriver

Dr. Samuel Tyriver, PT, DPT, CWC has spent over a decade treating patients whose pain defies conventional diagnosis. What began as clinical observation eventually became a framework: the Six Keys to Your Inner Pharmacy, refined through years of patient work and grounded in the latest pain science research. Determined to reach beyond his own practice, he founded the Certified Mindbody Trained Therapist™ program, training physical and occupational therapists across the country to treat chronic pain through the lens of the nervous system rather than tissue alone.

His central conviction has never wavered: your nervous system is not broken. It is only trying too hard to keep you safe.

Dr. Tyriver lives and practices in Milwaukee, Wisconsin.

Hayley DiMarco

Hayley DiMarco is a bestselling author and founder of Hungry Planet, a content and design studio, with more than fifty published titles. She writes from the inside of the experience this book describes: a nervous system that stayed on high alert long after the threat had passed. Her voice is confessional, direct, and honest about what it actually costs to live inside a body that has learned to be afraid. She shares about her life and field-tested theology at GodGirl.com.

Hayley lives with her husband Michael (another bestselling author) and their three dogs in Milwaukee, Wisconsin.

More resources

The conversation doesn't end here.

At OverprotectiveBrain.com you'll find answers to the most common questions about chronic pain and the nervous system, written in the same language as this book. You'll also find *The Overprotective Brain* podcast, where you can watch or listen to Dr. Samuel Tyriver and Hayley DiMarco go deeper each episode with the most common questions (and uncommon answers!) regarding pain, fear, and anxiety.

If something in these pages made something click, clicking the website is where you go next.

OverprotectiveBrain.com

www.ingramcontent.com/pod-product-compliance
Lightning Source LLC
LaVergne TN
LVHW100307210926
848480LV00003B/1047